Identifying and Measuring Alcoholic Personality Characteristics

W. Miles Cox, *Editor*

NEW DIRECTIONS FOR METHODOLOGY OF SOCIAL AND BEHAVIORAL SCIENCE

DONALD W. FISKE, *Editor-in-Chief*

Number 16, June 1983

Paperback sourcebooks in
The Jossey-Bass Social and Behavioral Science Series

Jossey-Bass Inc., Publishers
San Francisco • Washington • London

W. Miles Cox (Ed.)
Identifying and Measuring Alcoholic Personality Characteristics.
New Directions for Methodology of Social and Behavioral Science, no. 16.
San Francisco: Jossey-Bass, 1983.

New Directions for Methodology of Social and Behavioral Science Series
Donald W. Fiske, *Editor-in-Chief*

New Directions for Methodology of Social and Behavioral Science is published quarterly by Jossey-Bass Inc., Publishers. Subscriptions, single-issue orders, change of address notices, undelivered copies, and other correspondence should be sent to *New Directions* Subscriptions, Jossey-Bass Inc., Publishers, 433 California Street, San Francisco, California 94104.

Editorial correspondence should be sent to the Editor-in-Chief, Donald W. Fiske, University of Chicago, Chicago, Illinois 60637.

Library of Congress Catalogue Card Number LC 82-82178

International Standard Serial Number ISSN 0271-1249

International Standard Book Number ISBN 87589-964-1

Cover art by Willi Baum

Manufactured in the United States of America

Ordering Information

The paperback sourcebooks listed below are published quarterly and can be ordered either by subscription or single-copy.

Subscriptions cost $35.00 per year for institutions, agencies, and libraries. Individuals can subscribe at the special rate of $21.00 per year *if payment is by personal check.* (Note that the full rate of $35.00 applies if payment is by institutional check, even if the subscription is designated for an individual.) Standing orders are accepted. Subscriptions normally begin with the first of the four sourcebooks in the current publication year of the series. When ordering, please indicate if you prefer your subscription to begin with the first issue of the *coming* year.

Single copies are available at $7.95 when payment accompanies order, and *all single-copy orders under $25.00 must include payment.* (California, New Jersey, New York, and Washington, D.C., residents please include appropriate sales tax.) For billed orders, cost per copy is $7.95 plus postage and handling. (Prices subject to change without notice.)

Bulk orders (ten or more copies) of any individual sourcebook are available at the following discounted prices: 10–49 copies, $7.15 each; 50–100 copies, $6.35 each; over 100 copies, *inquire.* Sales tax and postage and handling charges apply as for single copy orders.

To ensure correct and prompt delivery, all orders must give either the *name of an individual* or an *official purchase order number.* Please submit your order as follows:

Subscriptions: specify series and year subscription is to begin.
Single Copies: specify sourcebook code (such as, MSBS8) and first two words of title.

Mail orders for United States and Possessions, Latin America, Canada, Japan, Australia, and New Zealand to:
Jossey-Bass Inc., Publishers
433 California Street
San Francisco, California 94104

Mail orders for all other parts of the world to:
Jossey-Bass Limited
28 Banner Street
London EC1Y 8QE

New Directions for Methodology of Social and Behavioral Science Series
Donald W. Fiske, *Editor-in-Chief*

MSBS1 *Unobtrusive Measurement Today,* Lee Sechrest
MSBS2 *Methods for Studying Person-Situation Interactions,* Lynn R. Kahle
MSBS3 *Realizations of Brunswik's Representative Design,* Kenneth R. Hammond, Nancy E. Wascoe
MSBS4 *Fallible Judgment in Behavioral Research,* Richard A. Shweder
MSBS5 *Quantitative Assessment of Research Domains,* Robert Rosenthal

MSBS6 *Issues in Aggregation,* Karlene H. Roberts, Leigh Burstein
MSBS7 *Biopolitics: Ethological and Physiological Approaches,* Meredith W. Watts
MSBS8 *Generalizing from Laboratory to Life,* Irwin Silverman
MSBS9 *Problems with Language Imprecision,* Donald W. Fiske
MSBS10 *Ethics of Human Subject Research,* Allan J. Kimmel
MSBS11 *Question Framing and Response Consistency,* Robin M. Hogarth
MSBS12 *Forms of Validity in Research,* David Brinberg, Louise H. Kidder
MSBS13 *Single-Case Research Designs,* Alan E. Kazdin, A. Hussain Tuma
MSBS14 *Using Observers to Study Behavior,* Donald P. Hartmann
MSBS15 *Naturalistic Approaches to Studying Social Interaction,* Harry T. Reis

Contents

Editor's Notes

Psychologists who work in the field of alcoholism no longer view the alcoholic personality as a viable concept, and it is not hard to see why this is so. The alcoholic personality, which originated in the medical model of alcoholism, is supposed to be a unique personality structure that accompanies the progressive and irreversible disease with which alcoholics are afflicted. Moreover, the essential elements of this structure are supposed to have been present in the alcoholic's premorbid personality and to have led inevitably to alcoholism. However, a scientific psychological investigation into the causes of alcoholism during the last two decades has led us to recognize that alcoholics are by no means a homogenous group, that there are multiple causes of alcoholism, and that the disease concept of alcoholism is untenable.

These observations are not meant to imply that the involvement of personality factors in alcoholism has been discarded as a legitimate object of study. To the contrary, the search for the alcoholic personality has been replaced by a more refined and elaborate view of how personality factors are involved in alcoholism. This issue of *New Directions for Methodology of Social and Behavioral Science* presents the new point of view, and it emphasizes the methodology by which alcoholics' personality characteristics can be identified and measured.

The first three chapters consider some global personality characteristics of alcoholics. In Chapter One, Miles Cox, Kin Lun, and Rodney Loper discuss the methodologies that have identified distinctive personality characteristics of alcoholics before the onset of alcoholism. The findings of the studies that they review point to some intriguing possibilities for the prevention of alcoholism. The authors also discuss some important new directions that future research should take in order better to delineate the personality precursors of alcoholism.

What happens when a person drinks alcohol after he or she has become alcoholic is the topic of Chapter Two. The body of research that James Langenbucher and Peter Nathan review clearly indicates that measurable changes in alcoholics' personality characteristics occur when they drink alcohol. Since these changes are not always desirable, they present some puzzling questions surrounding alcoholics' motivations for consuming alcohol. Such questions need to be answered by future studies that would overcome the design problems hampering prior research.

In Chapter Three, Damaris Rohsenow describes perceived control as one personality variable that pervades the lives of alcoholics. Their perceptions of the source of control in their lives are related both to the reasons why they drink and to their drinking-related problems. Moreover, such aspects of alcoholics' personalities as their styles of relating to other people, the type of treatment that they prefer, and the outcome of treatment can all be understood in terms of perceived control. Finally, Rohsenow suggests some ways in which clinicians can use alcoholics' perceived control to improve treatment effectiveness, and she indicates some directions that future research on this topic should take.

The remaining three chapters in this volume are concerned with ways in which alcoholics can be grouped to eliminate the distortions created by the view that alcoholics form a single homogenous group with respect to their personality characteristics. In Chapter Four, Carole Benson and Sharon Wilsnack review the literature that has identified differences between alcoholic men and women. These differences have been found to occur in a variety of personality variables, including the onset and course of alcoholism, concomitant and premorbid psychopathology, life experience risk factors, motivations for drinking, self-concept and self-esteem, and social role influences. The authors find that prior research is limited in a variety of ways, and they make some specific suggestions for the methodology and content of future studies.

In Chapter Five, Craig MacAndrew asks whether the vast amount of research that used the Minnesota Multiphasic Personality Inventory (MMPI) to study alcoholics can help to identify a single personality structure that is shared by alcoholics but not by other individuals. He concludes that neither a scale nor a profile approach can make the MMPI useful for this purpose. Instead, MacAndrew uses the MAC Alcoholism Scale from the MMPI to derive a taxonomy of drinkers' personalities that promises to be quite fruitful in future research on the etiology and course of alcoholism.

In Chapter Six, Douglas Jackson presents evidence that there are multiple types of alcoholic personalities. He reviews studies that identify a variety of types of psychopathology associated with alcoholism and describes one alternative to the traditional procedure of comparing mean differences between alcoholics and nonalcoholics on various personality measures. Jackson suggests a number of ways in which the existing research on alcoholic personalities could be improved. He focuses on the manner in which personality characteristics are measured and on procedures for analyzing the results of these studies.

Most of the chapters in this volume are based on a symposium entitled "The Alcoholic Personality and Its Measurement" that was presented at the eighty-eighth annual convention of the American Psychological Association in Montreal in August 1980. The general conclusion reached by symposium participants is reiterated here: There seems to be not one alcoholic personality but several, which can best be understood in terms of their interaction with other variables that help to explain alcoholism.

W. Miles Cox
Editor

W. Miles Cox is associate professor of psychology and director of the Drug Information Program at the University of Minnesota, Morris.

Preliminary research has narrowed the scope of studies aimed at finding personality precursors of alcoholism to the prospective longitudinal design.

Identifying Prealcoholic Personality Characteristics

W. Miles Cox
Kin-Shing Lun
Rodney G. Loper

Present approaches to obtaining an understanding of alcoholism stress the susceptibility of certain individuals to the pharmacological and psychological effects of alcohol. However, there seems to be little agreement about what causes an individual to be susceptible to these effects, although many explanations have been offered. Some investigators (Goodwin, 1979) search for genetic explanations and biochemical reactions to alcohol that might be inherited. Others emphasize environmental (Beigel and Ghertner, 1979) and sociocultural (Heath, 1976) influences. One of the variables that investigators looking for psychological explanations for vulnerability to alcoholism have emphasized is personality (Barnes, 1983; Williams, 1976). Nevertheless, psychologists seem increasingly to reject the notion that personality contributes to alcoholism. This trend stems in part from a misunderstanding of what is meant by alcoholic personality characteristics. The present chapter aims to clarify that misunderstanding.

There is much to be derived from the study of alcoholic personality characteristics, and we believe that the study of prealcoholic personality characteristics is an essential part of the endeavor. Our primary concern in this

W. M. Cox (Ed.). *Identifying and Measuring Alcoholic Personality Characteristics.* New Directions for Methodology of Social and Behavioral Science, no. 16. San Francisco: Jossey-Bass, June 1983.

chapter is with methodology for studying prealcoholic personality characteristics. We have two major goals: to delineate the types of methodology that the existing studies of prealcoholic personality characteristics have used and to point to some methodological considerations for future research on these characteristics.

Cox (1979) enumerated the potential benefits of identifying alcoholic personality characteristics. Some of these benefits have special relevance for the study of prealcoholic personality characteristics. Thus, identification of the personality antecedents of alcoholism would help considerably in clarifying the etiology of alcoholism, since it would allow us to determine the personal characteristics of persons who become dependent on alcohol and their motivations for doing so. More important, identifying antecedent alcoholic personality characteristics would help us to screen people who are at risk for alcoholism and to take measures that could prevent them from becoming alcoholic. Primary prevention techniques could have far-reaching consequences for reducing the human losses and suffering that surround the use of alcohol.

Ground Rules

Several basic assumptions need to be understood before we can decide whether antecedent alcoholic personality characteristics exist and describe what they are. First, Barnes (1979, 1980, 1983) has distinguished between clinical personality characteristics—those exhibited by alcoholics at the time of treatment—and prealcoholic personality characteristics. Although it is important to identify personality characteristics that distinguish alcoholics in treatment from nonalcoholics, we cannot assume that these characteristics were present before alcoholism developed. Instead of being the reasons for alcoholism, these personality characteristics may be consequences of alcoholism. It is essential to identify personality characteristics before the onset of alcoholism if we are to regard the characteristics as precursors of alcoholism.

Second, antecedent alcoholic personality characteristics are in themselves not sufficient to explain alcoholism. Instead, they must be considered together with other variables: genetic, environmental, and sociocultural influences. Surely, alcoholism results not from any one of these variables acting alone but from the interaction of all. Not only should prealcoholic personality characteristics not be taken as leading inevitably to alcoholism, they should not be interpreted as pejorative and pathological personality characteristics, as some writers have done. In fact, some prealcoholic personality characteristics might be considered socially desirable.

Third, failure to find a distinctive, unitary prealcoholic personality cluster does not necessarily mean that prealcoholic personality characteristics do not exist. Instead, the absence of a single cluster may simply reflect the heterogeneity of persons who become alcoholic. In this connection, we can note that different research methods produce different results. Recently, multivariate statistical techniques have been used to identify alcoholic personality subtypes that comparisons of mean differences of alcoholics and nonalcoholics have obscured. (See the chapter by Jackson in this volume.) Thus, it seems likely that these techniques can also be used to identify a variety of personality precursors of alcoholism that might otherwise go unrecognized.

Research Findings

What has research learned about prealcoholic personality characteristics? Many studies of prealcoholic personality characteristics have described their procedures as longitudinal. Since several different methods of study can be discerned, we prefer to refine this description. Thus, we distinguish between archival, archival longitudinal, and retrospective studies. We describe those three types in this section. In the following section, we describe the prospective longitudinal study. We believe that the prospective longitudinal study is ideal for identifying prealcoholic personality characteristics, although it has yet to be used in conducting a study.

Archival Studies. In the typical archival study, the investigator has access to data on subjects' personality characteristics that others collected many years earlier for purposes unrelated to alcoholic personality characteristics. The archival investigator first determines which subjects in the original study became alcoholic at a later point in their lives. He or she then analyzes the original data to determine whether the prealcoholics had personality characteristics that differed from those of the individuals who did not become alcoholic. We have identified four archival studies.

McCord and McCord (1960, 1962) utilized archival data from 255 boys followed in the Cambridge-Somerville (Massachusetts) Youth Study, which began in 1935 when the boys were an average of nine years old. The purpose of the Cambridge-Somerville study was to gather data on childrearing practices among the lower classes and to prevent delinquency. Between 1939 and 1945, social workers visited the homes of the boys and their families approximately twice a month. The observations recorded during these visits were the data on which McCord and McCord based their ratings of various personality characteristics. While McCord and McCord were making the personality ratings (between 1955 and 1957), they also examined various official community records to determine which of the boys had become alcoholic during adulthood. They found that twenty-nine of the subjects in the Cambridge-Somerville study met their criteria: membership in Alcoholics Anonymous, having presented oneself for treatment for alcoholism, or having been convicted of public drunkenness at least twice. Chi-square statistics comparing the boyhood personality ratings of the twenty-nine alcoholics with the ratings of 158 subjects who were neither alcoholics nor criminals indicated that prealcoholics had been more self-confident, aggressive, active, sadistic, fearless, and sexually anxious than other boys. McCord and McCord summarized this cluster of characteristics as overemphasis on masculinity, which they felt served to mask feminine, passive proclivities.

Robins and his associates (Robins, 1966; Robins and others, 1962) used records maintained on 367 male and 141 female children seen at a child guidance clinic in St. Louis between 1924 and 1929. Thirty years after they were treated at the clinic, the subjects were interviewed about their drinking practices and problems, and each subject was classified as an alcoholic, a heavy drinker, or one with no excessive drinking. Matched subjects (seventy males, twenty-nine females) were chosen from public school records in order to compare rates of future alcoholism for normal children and for children with behavior problems. Comparison indicated a higher rate of alcoholism for the clinic group (21 percent for males, 8 percent for females) than for the comparison group (3 percent for males, 0 percent for females), but prealcoholic personality characteristics could be assessed only for the clinic group, since there were no clinical records on the comparison group. Personality assessments of the clinic group evaluated each subject for thirty-five symptoms of antisocial behavior (such as running away, theft, assault) and for thirty-six symptoms of neurotic behavior (such as passivity, learning disabilities, poor coordination). No sex differences were reported, but chi-square analyses indicated that the proportion of alcoholics who exhibited a set of fifteen antisocial symptoms during childhood was significantly higher than the proportion of members of the other two groups of drinkers who exhibited the set. However, the neurotic symptoms were distributed according to chance among the three groups of drinkers. Thus, Robins' study substantiates the findings of McCord and McCord that antisocial personality characteristics predate alcoholism.

In Minnesota, Hoffmann and others (1974), Kammeier and others (1973), and Loper and others (1973) took advantage of the fact that the Minnesota Multiphasic Personality Inventory (MMPI) had been administered to entering freshmen in many colleges of the University of Minnesota from the late 1940s until 1962 as part of the admission procedure and used the MMPI records as their archival data to study prealcoholic personality characteristics. Before beginning the study, they searched patient files at two major alcoholism treatment centers in Minnesota, Hazelden Treatment Center and Willmar State Hospital (where the MMPI was administered to incoming patients), to determine whether alcoholic patients at these facilities had been students at the university. Thirty-two male patients who had MMPI records at the university. Thirty-two male patients who had MMPI records at the university were identified. Their mean age on the two occasions on which they had taken the MMPI—as college freshmen and as alcoholics in treatment—was 20.5 years and 33.5 years, respectively.

First, Kammeier and others (1973) compared the prealcoholic and treatment profiles and found that, although both profiles were elevated on the same scales, only the treatment profiles showed indications of maladjustment and distress. Then, to determine whether prealcoholic personality characteristics were evident in the earlier MMPI records, Loper and others (1973) compared these records with the MMPI records of 148 male classmates chosen at random, who presumably did not become alcoholics at a rate any higher than that observed in the general population. Analysis using *t* tests indicated that prealcoholics had significantly higher scores on three of the MMPI standard scales (*F, Pd,* and *Ma*) and on two of the Wiggins content scales (Authority Conflict and Poor Health), but there were no significant differences on two MMPI special scales that measured maladjustment. The researchers inferred that the prealcoholics were more impulsive, nonconforming, and gregarious than their peers, but they were not more maladjusted. Further, item analysis indicated that thirty-five items differentiated prealcoholics from classmates. Collectively, these items suggested that prealcoholics were less conventional, had more health concerns, and were more socially cynical and romantic than their classmates (Hoffmann, 1976). The thirty-five items to which prealcoholics responded True significantly more often than their classmates have not been published. We list their MMPI booklet numbers here: 12, 14, 25, 37, 53, 56, 64, 95, 106, 116, 117, 118, 124, 126, 131, 135, 200, 224, 230, 231, 272, 288, 294, 302, 322, 329, 348, 376, 422, 424, 435, 438, 481, 502, 521.

In a subsequent analysis of the data, Hoffmann and others (1974) compared prealcoholic and treatment responses to individual MMPI items and scores on the Wiggins content scales and various alcoholism scales. They also compared the prealcoholics and their classmates on the alcoholism scales. Results corroborated the profile analyses conducted by Kammeier and others (1973) in that the alcoholics were distinctly more maladjusted and distressed at the time of treatment than they were during college. Alcoholics in treatment also had significantly higher scores on four of the nine alcoholism scales than they had as freshmen. Finally and most importantly, the prealcoholics had significantly higher scores on the MacAndrew and Rosenberg alcoholism scales than their classmates did. The MacAndrew scale classified 72 percent of the prealcoholics as alcoholic, 72 percent of the classmates as nonalcoholic, and 56 percent of the alcoholics in treatment as alcoholic. The corresponding percentages for the Rosenberg scale were 72 percent, 72 percent, and 88 percent.

In summary, this research indicates that, although prealcoholics may not show symptoms of maladjustment and distress, they do have identifiable personality characteristics that distinguish them from control subjects. It is noteworthy that the Minnesota archival studies were the first to use a standardized personality inventory.

Vaillant and Milofsky (1982) analyzed data from a sample of 456 males who served as control subjects in a study of juvenile delinquency by Glueck and Glueck (1950, 1968) that began in 1940. Clearly, the Gluecks' method of study was longitudinal. However, Vaillant and Milofsky seem to have used only the childhood data from the Gluecks' subjects to assess prealcoholic personality characteristics, so we classify their study as archival, not archival longitudinal. The childhood data include social service records and records taken during interviews with the boys, their parents, and teachers. Instead of evaluating personality characteristics per se, Vaillant and Milofsky rated the subjects on such variables as childhood environmental weaknesses, poor infant health, and truancy and school behavior problems (that is, antisocial behavior). To determine the degree to which subjects experienced alcohol problems during adulthood, Vaillant and Milofsky rated the alcohol problems of 442 subjects on three different scales. Ratings were based on subjects' responses to questions about alcohol problems during interviews presumably conducted by Glueck and Glueck when the subjects were thirty-one and forty-seven years old. Seventy-one subjects were alcohol-dependent according to DSM-III, 110 were alcohol abusers according to Vaillant's Problem Drinking Scale, while the number of subjects who were alcoholic according to Cahalan's scale is not given.

Product-moment correlations indicated that all three premorbid variables named earlier, in addition to number of alcoholic relatives and absence of South European ethnicity, were significantly related to later alcohol problems. Nevertheless, Vaillant and Milofsky (1982) diminish the importance of antisocial behavior as a precursor of alcoholism by suggesting that antisocial behavior more often follows alcoholism than precedes it. Although their data indicate that only 3 percent of the variance in alcohol problems during adulthood can be explained by childhood antisocial behavior (that is, by school behavior problems), the data do not indicate when the adult subjects became either antisocial or alcoholic. Hence, the data that these researchers present do not allow us to conclude that antisocial behavior more frequently follows alcoholism than precedes it.

Archival Longitudinal Studies. The archival longitudinal study resembles the archival study in that it uses data collected on individuals before alcohol became a problem in their lives and compares these data with those from individuals for whom alcohol did not become a problem. The archival longitudinal study differs from the archival study in that it compares data collected at more than one point in the subjects' lifetime.

Jones's (1968, 1971) archival data were taken from the Oakland Growth Study, which began thirty years previously. The Oakland Growth Study followed a heterogeneous, middle-class sample of males and females closely from the age of ten and a half until graduation from high school and less closely during adulthood. The Oakland study recorded a variety of psychometric and observational data. Using these data and California *Q* set ratings and interpersonal *Q* sorts, Jones assessed fifty-two male and forty-five female subjects on 100 personality characteristics at three points during their lives: junior high school, senior high school, and adulthood. In addition, she used information about the quantity and frequency of alcohol consumption obtained from interviews with the subjects when they were thirty-eight years old to separate them into five categories of drinking behavior: abstainers, light drinkers, moderate drinkers, heavy drinkers, and problem drinkers.

For the male subjects (Jones, 1968), personality characteristics were reported only for the problem drinkers, moderate drinkers, and abstainers. Jones used *t* tests to compare the problem drinkers with the moderate drinkers and the problem drinkers with the abstainers. However, no overall test of significance was reported before the multiple t tests were undertaken. The results indicated that, in junior high school, the six problem drinkers were distinguished by uncontrolled impulsivity, extroversive behavior, rebelliousness, and overemphasis on masculinity. In contrast, the seventeen moderate drinkers and the two abstainers were characterized as overcontrolled, responsible, introversive, dependent, and submissive. In general, the same distinguishing personality characteristics of the three categories of drinkers were apparent during senior high school and adulthood.

Analysis of the data on female subjects (Jones, 1971) included comparisons among all five groups of drinkers. Statistical analysis again involved two-group comparisons, and although Jones reported results only as levels of significance, presumably the comparisons again involved computation of multiple t tests. Personality descriptions of the five categories were usually taken from the adult assessments, but, with a few exceptions, the adult descriptions were accurate for early adolescence as well. Unlike their male counterparts, the three problem drinkers and the four abstainers in Jones's female sample had personality characteristics in common that suggested inadequate coping devices. The members of both groups were described as pessimistic, withdrawn, and self-defeating and as less independent and less self-satisfied than the eighteen moderate drinkers. They also were judged to be sensitive to criticism, judgmental, and distrustful. However, there were some personality characteristics that abstainers and problem drinkers did not share, which might account for their different approaches to alcohol. That is, while the abstainers were conventional, consistent, responsible, and emotionally controlled, the problem drinkers exhibited unstable and unpredictable impulsivity. To account for these results, Jones hypothesized that the excessive drinking by problem drinkers was an attempt to cope with feelings of inadequacy and despondency, while the abstinence and the personality characteristics of the nondrinkers originated from adolescence and the adverse influence of their parents' drinking problems.

The twelve heavy drinkers in Jones's female sample were very different from both the problem drinkers and the moderate drinkers. As adolescents, they had been rated higher than members of the other groups on social skills, charm, and expressiveness, and they were described as power-oriented, self-satisfied, and self-indulgent. In adulthood, they were depicted as self-confident in social situations, and they seemed to use alcohol more for social than for compensatory reasons. Although the moderate drinkers were less socially oriented than the heavy drinkers, they were judged to be stable, productive individuals who had a satisfactory self-image. Finally, the eight light drinkers were described as the most responsible, fastidious, and overcontrolled of the forty-five female subjects. They were rated as more self-defeating and less socially skillful than the moderate drinkers but less vulnerable, less sensitive to criticism, and more socially skillful than the abstainers.

In summary, instead of finding personality differences between persons who did and did not become alcoholic, as researchers who pursued archival studies did, Jones (1968, 1971) related specific personality characteristics to various specific drinking behaviors. However, since some of the categories of drinking behavior that Jones studied had very small frequencies, the extent to which we can generalize her findings may be limited.

Retrospective Studies. Prealcoholic personality characteristics have sometimes been assessed by asking alcoholics in treatment, their families, or both to describe the alcoholics' personalities before they became alcoholic. We describe this type of study as retrospective in nature. While the personality descriptions that this type of study produces can be inaccurate due to distortions in memory, the retrospective study can nevertheless generate useful information, especially by helping to formulate hypotheses that can be tested with other types of designs. In addition, the findings of retrospective studies have generally been consistent with those of studies that use other methodology.

One example of retrospective assessment of premorbid personality is the "nature-nurture" study of alcoholism conducted by Goodwin and others (1975). Subjects were 133 Danish male adoptees ranging in age from twenty-three to forty-five. Fourteen were diagnosed as alcoholic by the researchers. Each subject was interviewed about his childhood personality characteristics. Chi-square statistics indicated that the alcoholics more frequently depicted themselves as exhibiting such antisocial and masculine personality characteristics as truancy, delinquency, disobedience to adults, hyperactivity, aggressiveness, and impulsivity during childhood than the nonalcoholics did. The alcoholics also more frequently reported themselves to have been shy, sensitive, and insecure than the nonalcoholics did, which suggests that the overt masculinity and aggressiveness of the alcoholics were a reaction against their underlying feelings.

A study by Tarter and others (1977) provides another example of alcoholics' retrospective accounts of their prealcoholic personality characteristics. The investigators compared the frequency with which various groups recalled having had, before age twelve, various characteristics that might indicate minimal brain dysfunction. The group of severe (primary) alcoholics included nine males and nine females, the group of less severe (secondary) alcoholics included twenty males and eight females, the group of nonalcoholic psychiatric patients included twenty-two males and twenty-seven females, and the group of "normal" controls included twenty males and seven females. There were no sex differences in the characteristics evaluated, but chi-square analyses indicated that the primary alcoholics more often recalled that they had been impulsive, easily frustrated, underachieving, and inclined not to complete projects during childhood than the members of other groups did.

Vaillant (1980) reported some analyses from a sample of 204 males on whom longitudinal study had begun while they were sophomores in college between 1940 and 1942. The subjects were studied closely while they were in college, then followed with biennial questionnaires and occasional interviews and other testing between the ages of twenty-two and fifty-eight. The subjects were chosen for their physical and psychological good health. The original intent of the study presumably was to determine whether and under what circumstances healthy men would develop physical and psychological maladies. However, it is unclear that an original intent was to study the precursors of alcoholism, and it is also unclear who the original investigators were.

The data analyses that Vaillant (1980) reports are both retrospective and contemporaneous, and our rationale for classifying his study as retrospective is that he used only retrospective data for his assessment of the precursors of alcoholism. That is, Vaillant's data were ratings (worst, intermediate, best)—based on retrospective judgments of various information obtained from home visits, developmental histories, and psychiatric interviews while the subjects were college students—of the subjects' "childhood environment." Judgments were made of the drinking status of the 184 subjects in the final sample on the basis of biennial questionnaires extending over thirty years. Forty-eight subjects were judged to have used alcohol little, ninety-two were classified as social users, sixteen as heavy social users, and twenty-eight as abusers or problem drinkers.

Inspection of the childhood data indicated that the problem drinkers were approximately equally represented in the three qualities of childhood environment, which suggests that alcoholism cannot be predicted by childhood environment. No significant relationships were found between the subjects' future alcohol use and the quality of their early relationships with their parents, childhood psychological problems, or psychological soundness in college. Unfortunately, these variables do not represent specific personality measures.

The one personality variable that Vaillant (1980) did study, oral dependency, was analyzed contemporaneously. That is, it occurred while the alcohol problems were developing. Vaillant reviewed the subjects' entire records to find objective vignettes that illustrated traits that he related to oral dependency: pessimism, passivity, self-doubt, fear of sex, suggestibility, and dependence. Although correlations between the number of vignettes and subjects' adult drinking status indicate a significant relationship, Vaillant (1980, p. 184) concluded that "the antecedents of orality and alcoholism were different, but once alcohol abuse had developed, oral vignettes were common." However, Vaillant neglects to present the data that allowed him to reach this conclusion.

Summary of Research Findings. There is a remarkable consistency in the findings of the nine studies that we have just reviewed. Although these studies used a variety of research methods and tested a variety of subjects, all except Vaillant's (1980) found evidence for prealcoholic personality characteristics. However, Vaillant did not include personality measures in his analyses of prealcoholics. The similarity of personality characteristics identified by the other eight studies is striking. Thus, the seven studies of males indicate that prealcoholic and problem drinking males have strong antisocial and masculine tendencies and poor impulse control. Researchers describe these individuals as delinquent, nonconforming, and rebellious; self-confident, independent, and aggressive; undercontrolled, hyperactive, and impulsive. The single study of problem drinking females (Jones, 1971) found that they were manipulative and self-defeating.

The studies did not fully explore the reasons why persons with these particular personality characteristics are more likely than others to develop problems with alcohol, but several possibilities are readily apparent. For example, the antisocial, masculine male in our society seems likely to overindulge in alcohol because overindulgence is antisocial and because it bolsters the image that a male has of himself as a man. Another likely possibility is that overindulgence in alcohol brings immediate gratification, and so it is a behavior that impulsive individuals, both male and female, frequently engage in with little regard for the long-range consequences. These and other possibilities need to be systematically investigated in future, prospective longitudinal studies.

Prospective Longitudinal Studies

The prospective longitudinal study, like the archival longitudinal study, examines the same subjects at periodic intervals over an extended period of time. Unlike the archival longitudinal study, the prospective longitudinal study follows a design and procedure worked out in advance of any actual data collection.

The prospective longitudinal study has one obvious advantage: It allows us to determine unequivocally whether the identified personality characteristics are antecedents or consequences of alcoholism. Future studies that adopt this design will need to consider three things in particular: the subject pool tested, the assessment instruments used, and the statistical procedures followed in analyzing the results. Future prospective longitudinal studies will be able to profit from archival, archival longitudinal, and retrospective studies by avoiding the pitfalls into which studies of these kinds have fallen and by being guided by the hypotheses that existing studies suggest.

Subjects. The studies of prealcoholic personality characteristics have not utilized random samples of subjects. For example, Robins's (Robins, 1966; Robins and others, 1962) subjects were patients at a guidance clinic during childhood, while the alcoholics studied by Kammeier, Hoffmann, and Loper (Kammeier and others, 1973; Hoffmann and others, 1974; Loper and others, 1973) were male inpatients in treatment facilities. In Vaillant's (1980) study, the individuals selected for study were specimens of physical and psychological good health. Thus, in none of these studies do we know whether the findings are peculiar to the particular alcoholics studied or whether they are true for alcoholics in general.

To circumvent this difficulty, future prospective longitudinal studies will have to test a wide variety of subjects. The information gained will allow us not only to assess how personality characteristics are related to a variety of patterns of alcohol use and abuse but also to identify what personality characteristics might protect a person from becoming alcoholic. To accomplish this end and to allow for the high rates of attrition that will inevitably occur, it will be necessary for future studies to test a very large number of subjects.

We believe that school systems would be an ideal source of subjects for future prospective longitudinal studies. Here, researchers would have access to a large, relatively stable body of subjects of both sexes representing a variety of sociocultural and ethnic backgrounds. Moreover, school systems have ongoing information-gathering mechanisms that could easily incorporate psychological assessments. The schools themselves would also stand to gain from these research efforts, which could eventually be used in preventive programs identifying students at risk for developing problems with alcohol.

As a matter of fact, one successful, prototypical data-gathering procedure in school systems, Project TALENT (Flanagan and others, 1964), already exists. This longitudinal data base includes some personality and value measures, but it was not designed to study alcoholism, and it does not include measures of drinking behavior. Nevertheless, this comprehensive longitudinal study could serve as a model for prospective longitudinal studies of prealcoholic personality characteristics that researchers will conduct in the future. More recently, a proposed thirty-year multidisciplinary longitudinal study on the etiology of alcoholism has been initiated at Rutgers University (Lester, personal communication, August 30, 1979).

Assessment. The procedure that most past studies of prealcoholic personality characteristics have followed involves rating subjects on various personality characteristics from the available observational, psychometric, and interview data recorded early in their lives. In contrast, future prospective longitudinal studies will have to conduct comprehensive assessments of personality in order to ensure that any personality variable that might conceivably antedate alcoholism will not be overlooked. Completeness is especially important for longitudinal studies because of the enormous expenditures of time and money that are necessary to conduct them.

One possible way of conducting a comprehensive assessment of personality is to use a well-established personality inventory, such as the MMPI. In fact, the MMPI is the psychometric instrument that has been used most frequently in existing studies of alcoholics (Cox, 1979). Its use in future prospective longitudinal studies would allow us to compare data from prealcoholics with data already collected from alcoholics and perhaps to disentangle the personality characteristics that are antecedents of alcoholism from the characteristics that are consequences of alcoholism. Although the efficacy of the MMPI for distinguishing alcoholics from nonalcoholics has been questioned (see the chapter by MacAndrew in this volume), it has been used quite productively in constructing typologies of alcoholics (see the chapters by Jackson and MacAndrew in this volume), and it seems likely that the MMPI would also be useful in constructing typologies of prealcoholics. In particular, use of the MAC

Alcoholism Scale for identifying prealcoholics is strongly recommended for future studies, especially in view of the findings of Sher and Levenson (1982).

Other promising personality inventories include the Differential Personality Inventory, the Personality Research Form, and the Sixteen Personality-Factor Questionnaire. All have been used for establishing alcoholic personality subtypes (Cox, 1979), and extension of this work to prealcoholics would undoubtedly be quite worthwhile. Another possibility for subtype identification is to administer more than one personality inventory to the same subjects, a procedure that has been followed successfully with alcoholics by Hoffmann and others (1975), Nerviano (1976), and Skinner and others (1974).

Improved assessments of subjects' alcohol use are also needed in future prospective longitudinal studies. Whereas the usual procedure in existing studies has been to dichotomize subjects as alcoholic or nonalcoholic in adulthood, future studies will need extensive data about subjects' patterns of alcohol use that can be organized into taxonomies and related to personality typologies. For readers who need more information on assessment of alcohol use, Skinner's (1981) comprehensive review of the basic principles and issues involved in the assessment of alcohol problems provides some excellent guidelines for organizing an assessment program. Moreover, Pattison and Kaufman (1982) offer multivariate procedures for assessing alcohol use and alcoholism as alternatives to the traditional binary diagnosis of a person as alcoholic or nonalcoholic. Finally, certain assessment instruments seem especially useful. For example, the Alcohol Use Inventory (Wanberg and others, 1977) yields scores on twenty-two scales that provide information about styles of alcohol use and favorable and unfavorable consequences of drinking. These scales can be plotted on a profile that provides an overall picture of an individual's alcohol use. The Drinking Profile (Marlatt, 1976) obtains information about drinking patterns and behavior, beverage preferences, and drinking rates and provides a behavioral assessment of alcoholism and problem drinking. This instrument has recently been revised (Marlatt and Miller, 1983).

In addition to personality measures and measures of drinking behavior, future prospective longitudinal studies will need measures of other variables that are likely to interact with personality to determine whether a person becomes alcoholic. For example, information will be needed about subjects' biochemical reactivity to alcohol, the environmental and sociocultural factors that influence patterns of alcohol consumption, and family history of alcoholism. A variety of demographic information will also be needed to provide the basis for subgroupings of subjects in multivariate analyses.

Statistical Analyses. As we indicated earlier, the statistical procedures that researchers use to evaluate prealcoholic personality characteristics depend on the manner in which they view the personality precursors of alcoholism. For the view that prealcoholics share a single cluster of personality characteristics, the appropriate research strategy is to compare the premorbid personalities of individuals who later in life become alcoholic with the early life personalities of persons who do not become alcoholic. This has been the usual strategy of the studies reviewed in this chapter. These studies have used simple, univariate statistical procedures—the *t* test and chi-square—to evaluate the observed personality differences between prealcoholic and control groups. In addition, some studies have used correlational techniques to assess the relationship between prealcoholic personality characteristics and the degree of alcohol abuse in later life. Although these research procedures have shown remarkable consistency in identifying some global personality characteristics that prealcoholics share, much valuable information about the personality precursors of alcoholism has almost certainly been obscured by using these univariate approaches, and for that reason they are not recommended for future research.

The alternative to viewing the personality precursors of alcoholism as a single cluster of characteristics is to construct a typology of prealcoholic personalities. To construct such a typology, statistical evaluation would have to use the same multivariate procedures that have been used to construct typologies of alcoholic personalities among alcoholics in treatment. While typological and cluster analyses may be useful techniques for delineating subgroups of prealcoholics, a word of caution is in order. Different computer programs for performing cluster analyses may generate subgroups differing in number and nature (see, for example, Thieret, 1982). Another useful technique for identifying personality characteristics of prealcoholics might be actuarial prediction in which a criterion (type and severity of alcoholism determined by objective measures) is specified, predictor variables (demographic data, personality profiles) are selected, and various mathematical techniques are used to determine the relationship between the configuration of predictor variables and the classification on the criterion. Readers who wish to become familiar with multivariate statistical procedures should consult the authors who have identified alcoholic personality subtypes as well as the writers on multivariate statistics who include Cooley and Lohnes (1962), Harris (1975), Nie and others (1975), and Van de Geer (1971).

Conclusions

Past studies of prealcoholic personality characteristics suffer from some notable deficiencies, including small, unrepresentative samples of subjects, incomplete assessments of personality and drinking behavior, and use of simple, univariate statistical procedures to compare prealcoholic and control groups. Despite these limitations, however, the prealcoholic personality characteristics identified by these studies are strikingly similar. Nevertheless, future prospective longitudinal studies, which we hope will succeed in establishing typologies of prealcoholic personalities, will need to give special consideration to the subjects who are tested, to the measurement instruments that are employed, and to the statistical procedures that are used in analyzing the results.

References

Barnes, G. E. "The Alcoholic Personality: A Reanalysis of the Literature." *Journal of Studies on Alcohol,* 1979, *40,* 571–634.

Barnes, G. E. "Clinical and Prealcoholic Personality Characteristics." In B. Kissin and H. Begleiter (Eds.), *The Biology of Alcoholism.* Vol. 6. *The Pathogenesis of Alcoholism: Psychosocial Factors.* New York: Plenum, 1983.

Barnes, G. E. "Characteristics of the Clinical Alcoholic Personality." *Journal of Studies on Alcohol,* 1980, *41,* 894–910.

Beigel, A., and Ghertner, S. "Toward a Social Model: An Assessment of Social Factors Which Influence Problem Drinking and Its Treatment." In B. Kissin and H. Begleiter (Eds.), *The Biology of Alcoholism.* Vol. 5. *Treatment and Rehabilitation of the Chronic Alcoholic.* New York: Plenum, 1979.

Cooley, W. W., and Lohnes, P. R. *Multivariate Procedures for the Behavioral Sciences.* New York: Wiley, 1962.

Cox, W. M. "The Alcoholic Personality: A Review of the Evidence." In B. A. Maher (Ed.), *Progress in Experimental Personality Research.* Vol. 9. New York: Academic Press, 1979.

Flanagan, J. C., and others. *Project TALENT: The American High School Student.* Pittsburgh: Project TALENT Office, University of Pittsburgh, 1964.

Glueck, S., and Glueck, E. *Unraveling Juvenile Delinquency.* New York: The Commonwealth Fund, 1950.

Glueck, S., and Glueck, E. *Delinquents and Nondelinquents in Perspective.* Cambridge, Mass.: Harvard University Press, 1968.

Goodwin, D. W., and others. "Alcoholism and the Hyperactive Child Syndrome." *Journal of Nervous and Mental Disease,* 1975, *160,* 349–353.

Goodwin, D. W. "Genetic Determinants of Alcoholism." In J. H. Mendelson and N. K. Mello (Eds.), *The Diagnosis and Treatment of Alcoholism.* New York: McGraw-Hill, 1979.

Harris, R. J. *A Primer of Multivariate Statistics.* New York: Academic Press, 1975.

Heath, D. B. "Anthropological Perspectives on the Social Biology of Alcohol: An Introduction to the Literature." In B. Kissin and H. Begleiter (Eds.), *The Biology of Alcoholism.* Vol. 4. *Social Aspects of Alcoholism.* New York: Plenum, 1976.

Hoffmann, H. "Personality Measurement for the Evaluation and Prediction of Alcoholism." In R. E. Tarter and A. A. Sugerman (Eds.), *Alcoholism: Interdisciplinary Approaches to an Enduring Problem.* Reading, Mass.: Addison-Wesley, 1976.

Hoffmann, H., Jackson, D. N., and Skinner, H. A. "Dimensions of Psychopathology Among Alcoholic Patients." *Journal of Studies on Alcohol,* 1975, *36,* 825–837.

Hoffmann, H., Loper, R. G., and Kammeier, M. L. "Identifying Future Alcoholics with MMPI Alcoholism Scales." *Quarterly Journal of Studies on Alcohol,* 1974, *35,* 490–498.

Jones, M. C. "Personality Correlates and Antecedents of Drinking Patterns in Adult Males." *Journal of Consulting and Clinical Psychology,* 1968, *32,* 2–12.

Jones, M. C. "Personality Antecedents and Correlates of Drinking Patterns in Women." *Journal of Consulting and Clinical Psychology,* 1971, *36,* 61–69.

Kammeier, M. L., Hoffmann, H., and Loper, R. G. "Personality Characteristics of Alcoholics as College Freshmen and at Time of Treatment." *Quarterly Journal of Studies on Alcohol,* 1973, *34,* 390–399.

Loper, R. G., Kammeier, M. L., and Hoffmann, H. "MMPI Characteristics of College Freshmen Males Who Later Become Alcoholics." *Journal of Abnormal Psychology,* 1973, *82,* 159–162.

Marlatt, G. A. "The Drinking Profile: A Questionnaire for the Behavioral Assessment of Alcoholism." In E. J. Mash and L. G. Terdal (Eds.), *Behavior Therapy Assessment: Diagnosis, Design, and Evaluation.* New York: Springer, 1976.

Marlatt, G. A., and Miller, W. R. *The Comprehensive Drinker Profile.* Odessa, Fla.: Psychological Assessment Resources, 1983.
McCord, W., and McCord, J. *Origins of Alcoholism.* Stanford, Calif.: Stanford University Press, 1960.
McCord, W., and McCord, J. "A Longitudinal Study of the Personality of Alcoholics." In D. J. Pittman and C. R. Snyder (Eds.), *Society, Culture, and Drinking Patterns.* New York: Wiley, 1962.
Nerviano, V. J. "Common Personality Patterns Among Alcoholic Males: A Multivariate Study." *Journal of Consulting and Clinical Psychology,* 1976, *44,* 104–110.
Nie, N. H., and others. *Statistical Package for the Social Sciences.* (2nd ed.) New York: McGraw-Hill, 1975.
Pattison, E. M., and Kaufman, E. *Encyclopedic Handbook of Alcoholism.* New York: Gardner Press, 1982.
Robins, L. N. *Deviant Children Grown Up: A Sociological and Psychiatric Study of Sociopathic Personality.* Baltimore, Md.: Williams & Wilkins, 1966.
Robins, L. N., Bates, W. M., and O'Neal, P. "Adult Drinking Patterns of Former Problem Children." In D. J. Pittman and C. R. Snyder (Eds.), *Society, Culture, and Drinking Patterns.* New York: Wiley, 1962.
Sher, K. J., and Levenson, R. W. "Risk for Alcoholism and Individual Differences in the Stress-Response-Dampening Effect of Alcohol." *Journal of Abnormal Psychology,* 1982, *91,* 350–367.
Skinner, H. A. "Assessment of Alcohol Problems: Basic Principles, Critical Issues, and Future Trends." In Y. Israel and others (Eds.), *Research Advances in Alcohol and Drug Problems.* Vol. 6. New York: Plenum, 1981.
Skinner, H. A., Jackson, D. N., and Hoffmann, H. "Alcoholic Personality Types: Identification and Correlates." *Journal of Abnormal Psychology,* 1974, *83,* 658–666.
Tarter, R. E., McBride, H., Buonpane, N., and Schneider, D. U. "Differentiation of Alcoholics." *Archives of General Psychiatry,* 1977, *34,* 761–768.
Thieret, N. L. "An Application of Four Cluster Analytic Methods to the Minnesota Multiphasic Personality Inventory in a Psychiatric Population." Doctoral dissertation, University of Minnesota, 1982.
Vaillant, G. E. "Natural History of Male Psychological Health. VIII: Antecedents of Alcoholism and 'Orality.'" *American Journal of Psychiatry,* 1980, *137,* 181–186.
Vaillant, G. E., and Milofsky, E. S. "The Etiology of Alcoholism: A Prospective Viewpoint." *American Psychologist,* 1982, *37,* 494–503.
Van de Geer, J. P. *Introduction to Multivariate Analysis for the Social Sciences.* San Francisco: W. H. Freeman, 1971.
Wanberg, K. W., Horn, J. L., and Foster, F. M. "A Differential Assessment Model for Alcoholism." *Journal of Studies on Alcohol,* 1977, *38,* 512–543.
Williams, A. F. "The Alcoholic Personality." In B. Kissin and H. Begleiter (Eds.), *The Biology of Alcoholism.* Vol. 4. *Social Aspects of Alcoholism.* New York: Plenum, 1976.

W. Miles Cox is associate professor of psychology and director of the Drug Information Program at the University of Minnesota, Morris.

Kin-Shing Lun is a research consultant at the Family Renewal Center, Fairview/Southdale Hospital, an outpatient facility for families with chemical dependency and sexual abuse problems in Edina, Minnesota.

Rodney G. Loper is a clinician in the Student Counseling Bureau and professor of psychology and health care psychology, University of Minnesota, Minneapolis.

Although human alcohol research is subject to many errors in the design of experiments and in the synthesis of results, recent work in this and related fields may point the way to a more stable, less conflicted body of knowledge.

The "Wet" Alcoholic: One Drink . . . Then What?

James Langenbucher
Peter E. Nathan

Our concern in this chapter is with the effects of beverage alcohol on the personalities of alcoholics. On the theoretical side, we do not mean to paint yet another picture of the alcoholic personality, nor do we mean to detail what the consumption of alcohol can do to a person unlucky enough to have an alcoholic personality. Sarason (1966, p. 15) reminds us that personality is "an area of investigation rather than an entity, real or hypothetical." Similarly, we do not wish to invest much effort in a critique of the alcoholic personality and the conceptual scheme—the unitary disease model of alcoholism—on which it is based. This model has received considerable attention (Caddy, 1978; Mello, 1975; Pattison, 1976). It holds that alcoholic individuals differ from normal individuals in psychological predisposition, nutritional status, or allergic sensitivity to alcohol; that these differences lead to psychological changes, biochemical changes, or both, which are progressive, irreversible, and predisposing to the experience of craving and loss of control; and that alcoholism can be remedied only by lifelong abstinence. It is our belief that research will benefit from a sensitivity to alternative approaches, such as that displayed by Pattison and others (1977), who view alcohol abuse and dependence as syndromes in a continuum of pathology. The syndromes are variable over time, they are the product of many factors, and they are inextricably bound up with other features of living.

W. M. Cox (Ed.). *Identifying and Measuring Alcoholic Personality Characteristics.* New Directions for Methodology of Social and Behavioral Science, no. 16. San Francisco: Jossey-Bass, June 1983.

On the methodological side, like Pihl and Spiers (1978, p. 98), we view personality as "a global concept, Lewinian in scope, eclectic in method, and probabilistic in prediction." We shall discuss not only studies of the effect of alcohol on alcoholics' responses to formal psychological tests, schedules, and inventories, but other, more influential studies that use soft dependent measures, including the effects on alcoholics' social behaviors (McNamee and others, 1968), subjective mood (Mendelson and others, 1964), fantasy production (Wolin and Mello, 1973), and still more transient emotional states.

Overview

Despite the objections to the unitary disease model of alcoholism, it has exerted a strong influence on study of the effects of alcohol on alcoholics. It is partially a function of its prevailing influence that our field has such a brief history—less than two decades. Into the 1960s, professional and community opinion, which was largely shaped by the unitary disease model, strongly opposed the administration of alcohol to alcoholics even for experimental purposes (Adesso, 1980).

Of equal authority in the development of our field has been Conger's (1956) tension reduction hypothesis—the idea that alcoholics drink because they have been negatively reinforced for doing so in the face of life stress. The tension reduction hypothesis has been influential in two ways. First, it has acted synergistically with the unitary disease model to direct the attention of researchers to the endogenous component of problem drinking, namely the alcohol-alcoholic interaction. It is because of the tension reduction hypothesis and the unitary disease model that the effects of alcohol on alcoholics' personalities seem to be so important. In contrast, other substance abuse problems have been conceptualized on the interpersonal, reference group, and even societal levels.

Second, the tension reduction hypothesis has led us to assume that only certain effects of alcohol are important, namely its effects on mood and affect. In contrast, the influence of alcohol on alcoholics' social relationships, marital interactions, and overt behavior has received little attention. Thus, the tension reduction hypothesis and the unitary disease model have served not only to guide the scope of research but also to limit it.

Programs of Study

We will refer throughout our discussion to the two major strategies that have been developed to study the effects of alcohol on alcoholics. The most influential studies are those of the chronic administration or prolonged drinking type. Here, volunteers from correctional or treatment facilities are restricted to a structured environment for long periods, with alcohol consumption controlled and dependent measures taken. Chronic administration researchers, who were most productive during the 1960s and early 1970s, have gathered data from live-in subjects over periods as long as ten weeks (Tamerin and others, 1970).

The other major type of experiment, the acute administration study, is generally conducted by researchers who lack live-in facilities. Here, subjects experience only one or two drinking sessions, in either a laboratory (Vannicelli, 1972) or a naturalistic setting (Williams, 1966, whose subjects were "heavy drinkers"). While subjects in these studies cannot be exposed to drinking schedules approximating those in vivo, such as a week-long drinking bout, they do not need to be provided with room and board for long periods, and thus samples in acute studies can be much larger than samples in chronic studies.

We note that two prominent hypotheses concerning the patterns and consequences of alcoholics' drinking have been tested in chronic and acute studies. These hypotheses are that alcoholics drink in order to reduce tension and that contact with alcohol sets up a process of craving (Jellinek, 1960), the response to which—drinking—is characterized by loss of control (Glatt, 1967; Jellinek, 1960). We now turn to a discussion of these and other findings.

Affective Change

As a sedative-hypnotic agent, ethanol is similar to the barbiturates and benzodiazepines. Each produces, in different ways, a temporary and nonspecific depressant effect on the central nervous system. Following Conger's (1956) tension reduction hypothesis, the effects of alcohol on alcoholics' affective, mood, and dispositional tendencies have been studied to determine whether a reduction of tension does in fact follow drinking.

Mood change following drinking has been a focus of both chronic and acute studies, which have used both scheduled and free-choice styles of drink administration. Chronic studies conducted by Mendelson and his colleagues (McGuire and others, 1966; McNamee and others, 1968; Mendelson and others, 1964; Tamerin and others, 1970) generally showed a negative and fairly linear dose response function. As blood alcohol level (BAL) rose, mood decayed. Some acute studies (Mayfield, 1968b; Vanderpool, 1969; van der Spuy, 1972) found a similar linear and negative relationship between BAL and self-reported mood.

Interestingly, two other acute studies (Mayfield, 1968a; Mayfield and Allen, 1967), both of which used intravenous alcohol drip procedures to control for expectancy effects, and Mueller (1965) also found a linear dose response function, but it was in the opposite direction. Alcohol produced elevated (or at least palliative) mood changes in alcoholic subjects. In another acute study, Vannicelli (1972) reported mixed findings. Most of her thirty alcoholic subjects became more depressed with increasing BAL, but only half reported more anxiety. In a natural party experiment with problem drinkers, Williams

(1966) found an inverted U-shaped dose response curve. He noticed positive mood changes in his subjects after a dose of about four ounces of beverage alcohol, but the effect reversed to marked anxiety and depression after sustained ad libitum drinking. Results from five chronic studies (Davis, 1971; Menaker, 1967; Nathan and O'Brien, 1971; Nathan and others, 1970; Tamerin and Mendelson, 1969) suggest a similar parabolic function. All these researchers noted brief euphoria in some subjects at the beginning of a drinking phase, followed by deterioration of mood as drinking progressed. Finally, one chronic study (Tracey and Nathan, 1976) found no change on multiple mood scales in four female alcoholics during a twelve-day drinking period.

In summary, acute studies have shown widely differing relationships between BAL and mood—positive linear, negative linear, parabolic, and mixed. The chronic studies have been more uniform, with subjects generally reporting a decay in mood as drinking progressed. In some cases, however, there was a brief euphoric period at the beginning of drinking, although one chronic study found no relationship between BAL and mood. Nevertheless, the true state of affairs may not be as chaotic as the accumulated results suggest. Studies have varied widely with regard to how subjects were selected; how long a time they were restricted to an unfamiliar, institutional, and potentially dysphoric experimental setting; whether alcohol was given orally or intravenously and by schedule or on demand; the types of dependent measures taken; and whether data were reported informally (as in most chronic studies) or subjected to rigorous statistical analysis (as in the acute studies). This lack of uniformity in experimental procedures may have yielded a needlessly mixed message.

Change in Self-Concept

Both clinical reports and personality studies of hospitalized alcoholics suggest that alcoholics drink to insulate themselves from feelings of low self-worth. This idea has inspired some experimental work. Vanderpool (1969) reported sophisticated analyses of responses to items compiled from two self-concept scales, the Tennessee Self-Concept Scale and an adjective checklist. The items were administered pre- and postexperimentally to two groups of fifty alcoholics each. Members of one group remained abstinent, while members of the other group drank to two dose levels—an interview-determined "optimal" level and one half of that amount. Contrary to expectation, the self-concept of the drinking alcoholics deteriorated on four dimensions—self-esteem, self-confidence and self-acceptance, adequacy, and social worth and tolerance for stress—and it showed no change on the fifth dimension, immaturity-insecurity.

Vanderpool's findings have been contradicted by both a chronic and an acute study. In the acute study, Berg (1971) administered two self-concept scales, the Chicago *Q* Sort and an adjective checklist, to twenty alcoholics and twenty matched controls, both before and after administration of alcohol. Both measures revealed positive shifts in the alcoholics on the self-ideal discrepancy scale from the Chicago *Q* Sort and on six scales from the adjective checklist at an average peak BAL of 132 mg/%. Virtually opposite shifts were noted in the control group at a lower peak BAL of 60 mg/%. These findings are consistent with some informal reports from the chronic study by McGuire and others (1966), which indicated increased self-esteem in some alcoholic subjects during prolonged drinking.

In summary, just as we saw in the studies of affective change in alcoholics, the studies of shifts in alcoholics' self-concepts after drinking reveal a conflicting pattern of results. However, the difficulty in measuring the hypothetical construct self-concept is an obstacle in such studies. Different researchers have chosen different instruments to measure self-concept. Some have devised measures of their own by combining items from existing self-concept scales. In addition, alcohol administration procedures have varied widely across these studies. It is not surprising that such heterogeneous procedures should fail to produce uniform results.

Changes in Fantasy Production

Few studies have examined the effects of alcohol on alcoholics' production of fantasies, and even these few have not focused on the same indexes of fantasy. For example, some have studied the effects of alcohol on dreams and hallucinations (Gross and others, 1971; Wolin and Mello, 1973), while others have examined responses to projective tests (Cutter and others, 1973; Key and others, 1972). These studies have related fantasies to such phenomena as drinking-induced drive for power (Cutter and others, 1973) and suppresion by alcohol of REM sleep and the possible implications of such suppression for alcoholic hallucinosis and withdrawal syndromes.

A chronic study by Wolin and Mello (1973) found that the frequency with which fourteen male alcoholics reported having dreams increased during prolonged drinking. However, no effect of BAL on REM activity was evident. Hallucinatory episodes occurred not only during withdrawal (consistent with clinical lore); they also occurred in two subjects at the beginning of drinking and at frequent intervals thereafter. Johnson and others (1970) found that hallucinations occurred among nonabstinent alcoholics, although others (Gross and others, 1971) have found no evidence for this.

The projective test that has generally been used to study the fantasy productions of alcoholics is the Thematic Apperception Test (TAT). For example, Cutter, Key, and colleagues (Key and others, 1972; Cutter and others, 1973) studied the TAT protocols of alcoholics in acute drinking studies designed to test McClelland's (McClelland and others, 1972) hypothesis that problem drinkers have an accentuated need for personalized power that is satisfied by alcohol, while only the social power needs of normal drinkers respond to alcohol. Contrary to McClelland's hypothesis, these studies found that power fantasies increased after the administration of alcohol for both types.

Changes in Desire for Alcohol (Craving and Loss of Control)

Craving. Craving for alcohol is generally viewed as an appetitive drive or "irresistible demand" (Jellinek, 1960, p. 140) to consume alcohol. In the "wet" alcoholic, the sensation of craving that accompanies the onset of partial withdrawal is relieved by continued drinking. Thus, craving as a correlate of physical dependence on alcohol has been used to explain the maintenance of excessive consumption within a single drinking bout.

Some information has been gathered on the induction of craving during drinking experiments with alcoholics. For example, Davis (1971) elicited self-reports from alcoholics undergoing experimental intoxication and found no support for craving. However, other researchers sensitive to the recent multivariate conceptualization of craving as a "system of interrelated responses involving subjective, physiological, behavioral, and biochemical components" (Hodgson and others, 1979, p. 380) have used various behavior indexes of craving. For example, Funderbunk and Allen (1977) required subjects to work for a reduction in the amount of time remaining before an upcoming drinking session. Some of the subjects appeared to manifest craving. Hodgson and others (1979) administered a priming dose of alcohol to alcoholic subjects, then measured the speed with which a subsequent criterion dose was consumed. They found that craving was induced only in severely alcoholic-dependent subjects. In our own laboratory (Nathan and others, 1980) we used a choice procedure to study the induction of craving. Two alcoholic subjects received a priming dose (alcohol or a placebo) via a double-blind procedure early each day, then chose between a moderate amount of alcohol given on demand or a large dose given after a long delay. Whether the priming dose contained alcohol or not, irresistible demand for alcohol (that is, craving) was never observed. For a period of twenty-eight days, the subjects invariably chose to receive the large dose, which they received after a delay of eight hours or more. In summary, the veridicality of the craving construct is uncertain at this point.

Loss of Control. Closely related to craving is the hypothetical construct of loss of control—the alcoholic's supposed inability to curb alcohol consumption once it has commenced. Loss of control has been described by Jellinek (1960) and others as a loss of freedom over drinking, an obsessive pursuit of alcohol accompanied by anxiety and panic in the face of encroaching withdrawal symptoms.

Loss of control has received much attention from researchers, but only one study (Ludwig and others, 1974) has provided even equivocal support for this construct. These investigators gave different priming doses of alcohol to alcoholics in the presence or absence of environmentally salient alcohol cues, then measured the rates at which subjects worked to earn more alcohol. High response rates, which the authors viewed as evidence for loss of control, were observed but only in the low-priming-dose, cues-present condition.

We know of no other study, acute or chronic, in which loss of control has been observed. Rather, alcoholics cease drinking in response to an interpersonal stress (Mendelson and Mello, 1966) or an offer of social or monetary reward, even after having been primed with a small dose of alcohol (Cohen and others, 1971). Both studies in which operant responding is required to earn alcohol (Mello and others, 1968) and studies in which free access to alcohol is allowed (Mello and Mendelson, 1971) have failed to report uncontrolled drinking by either male or female alcoholics. Instead, maintenance drinking to sustain moderate BALs has been observed in both male (Mello and Mendelson, 1971) and female alcoholics (Tracey and Nathan, 1976). In males, a biphasic pattern—several days of abstinent working to earn alcohol, followed by shorter periods in which the accumulated store is consumed—has also been observed (Nathan and others, 1970). In summary, the patterns of alcoholic drinking are consistent in that "wet" alcoholics show considerable control over their consumption.

Changes in Disposition to Behave

Just as the tension reduction hypothesis implicates the depressant effects of alcohol in the relief from anxiety that follows drinking, the disinhibition hypothesis holds that the depressant effects of alcohol act on the cerebral cortex to release certain (often undesirable) behaviors from inhibitory control (Adesso, 1980). The effects of alcohol on alcoholics' social and sexual behavior, aggression, and marital and familial functioning have been studied.

That drinking increases alcoholics' social behavior, or their desire for it, has been found in chronic studies designed to test the reinforcement values of social versus monetary rewards (Tracey and Nathan, 1976) as well as incidentally in other chronic (Mendelson and others, 1964) and acute (Diethelm and Barr, 1962) studies. The picture is mixed, however, since some chronic studies (Nathan and O'Brien, 1971) have reported decreases in the social motivation of alcoholics during drinking.

The connection between drinking and sexual fantasy and behavior in alcoholics remains relatively unexplored, although at least three such studies have been reported so far. Tamerin and Mendelson (1969) found increases in self-reported and staff-observed sexual interest in four male alcoholics during twenty-one days of drinking. Using a modified *Q* sort as their dependent variable, Tamerin and others (1970) found increased sexual interest in thirteen male alcoholics during fourteen to sixty days of drinking, despite subjects' expectation that sexual responses would be inhibited by alcohol. Eight male alcoholic subjects exposed by Wilson and others (1978) to erotic stimuli at peak BALs of up to 118 mg/% experienced inhibited sexual arousal (as measured by penile tumescence), particularly at high doses. Wilson has replicated this finding with social drinkers. Thus, alcohol seems consistently to inhibit physiological sexual arousal. Wilson and Lawson (1976) interpreted subjective sexual arousal in male social drinkers as a learned expectancy effect and controlled for expectancy via the balanced placebo design (described later in this chapter). Results indicated that it is the expectation of having received alcohol, not its actual presence in a drink, that initiates drinking-induced sexual arousal in male social drinkers.

Despite the frequent connection of alcohol to interpersonal conflict, we know of no study in which the effects of alcohol on alcoholics' aggressive impulses have been of more than peripheral interest or which has observed a consistent pattern of results. A major problem of experimental design in this area has been the reliance on analogues of aggression or on self-report indexes (for example, hostility), which need not covary with overt, in vivo behavior (for example, physical assault). These and other issues have been addressed by Adesso (1980) and by Carpenter and Armenti (1972).

One recent line of research has studied the effects of alcohol on alcoholics' marital and family relationships, usually during a conjoint hospitalization of alcoholics and their families during which alcohol is available. These studies are generally marked by extensive, idiographic assessments of subjects and their families and more recently by the use of formal interpersonal rating systems, such as the Coding Scheme for Interpersonal Conflict, and self-report instruments. Keenly sensitive to problems of external validity, Steinglass (1979) has allowed live-in subjects to design their own living quarters and to shop for food and prepare their own meals. However, internal validity has suffered: The manipulation, or even the simple monitoring, of key variables (such as alcohol consumption rates) was lacking, and results were presented in a highly interpretive mode.

Steinglass (1979) argued that drinking has a stabilizing influence on relationships within a family that has alcoholic members. In contrast, Billings and others (1979), who conducted the only acute study in this area, focused on alcoholic couples' problem-solving behaviors and found no effect for alcohol on the couples' interactional styles. But this study, like that of Steinglass, was hampered by manipulation problems: Half of the couples abstained from ad libitum drinking, and the average BAL of the alcoholic drinkers was only 26 mg/%.

In regard to treatment goals, then, a growing interest in family and marital factors accompanied by imaginative experimental designs with good external validity augurs well for the conduct of our enterprise. However, experimental attention to phenomena with forensic significance, such as the effects of alcohol on aggression and sexual expression, is diminishing.

Critique and Suggestions

Sample Integrity. Methodological reviews often point to the importance of thorough documentation of research subjects' degree of alcohol-related impairment, and Miller (1976) reviewed no fewer than ten alcoholism screening devices available at that time. However, we know of no study of the effects of alcohol on alcoholics' personality characteristics that has reported scores on such an instrument. Rather, informal indications of drinking history, along with a few demographic data, are the norm. While such information is useful, we feel that a quantitative estimate, via a specialized screening device, of each subject's involvement with alcohol must accompany research reports. Work by Skinner (1981) suggests that the Michigan Alcoholism Screening Test and the Alcohol Use Inventory yield reliable estimates of degree of impairment that are relatively free of response style biases and that have good concurrent and construct validity. We urge that they be used in future research.

Within-Sample Variability. A host of stable subject characteristics, including sex, age, education, and socioeconomic status, are often mentioned in research reports. Other characteristics, such as intelligence and marital status, should also be reported, but they rarely are. Additional, transient subject characteristics, including anxiety, arousal to perform a task, disposition to produce distorted or socially desirable responses, and expectancy effects have been implicated in differential human responses to alcohol. Researchers must make some attempt to report and control for these variables. Finally, gender differences in response to alcohol are important; see the chapter by Benson and Wilsnack in this volume.

Assessment of Blood Alcohol Level. Most acute studies have reported BALs achieved during an experiment, but some (Mueller, 1965; Williams, 1966) have paid little attention to the BAL or to the actual dose of alcohol consumed. Chronic researchers seem to have a generally poorer record of attention to this critical variable. For example, Mendelson and others (1964) gave standard, incremental doses of alcohol to ten male alcoholics during twenty-four days of drinking but never took BAL readings of their subjects. McNamee and others (1968) took BAL readings, but they omitted them from their research report.

If we are to make sense of the effects of alcohol on alcoholics' moods, sociability, sexual fantasies, and other phenomena, we must know how intoxicated subjects were when the measurements of these dependent variables were taken. Indeed, Maisto and others (1978) argue that objective and subjective effects of alcohol vary as a function of beverage type, speed of drinking, and position on the ascending or descending limb of the BAL curve. Clearly, future reports must provide BAL data, including which limb of the BAL curve subjects were on at the time of measurement. Toward this end, Nathan and others (1970) presented daily plots of subjects' breath alcohol levels, and Tracey and Nathan (1976) reported four daily breathalyzer readings as well as BAL values estimated hourly via on-line computer. For instances in which breath sampling is regarded as too reactive, Matthews and Miller (1979) have published two computer programs that estimate BALs from data on sex, body weight, and amount and rate of consumption. Such estimates are accurate to within about 10 mg/% —accuracy that is almost as good as that obtained with breath-testing methods.

Subject Tolerance of Alcohol. Tolerance of a dose of alcohol is at least a tripartite construct, consisting of innate or initial sensitivity to alcohol as well as of dose-induced changes in sensitivity acquired after both acute and chronic drinking episodes. Despite the importance of tolerance, we know of no study, chronic or acute, that has attempted to assess subjects' tolerance. In regard to sample integrity (that is, whether researchers employed truly alcohol-involved—and therefore alcohol-tolerant—subjects in their experiments), it is disturbing that many of the studies that we have reviewed report "obvious" signs of intoxication even at modest BALs (for example, 60 mg/% in Mayfield and Allen, 1967). Rough estimates of chronic tolerance can be obtained with the alcoholism screening devices mentioned earlier. Measurement of acute tolerance has also come within our grasp: The human liver retains markers of recent drinking (and thus, presumably, of acute tolerance) in the form of temporary alterations in enzymatic activity. It is now possible to estimate recent alcohol intake from the value of a single blood fraction, the level of serum gamma-glutamyl transpeptidase (GGTP). Thus, researchers can now estimate pre-experimental acute tolerance of alcohol in their experimental subjects.

In addition to pre-experimental tolerance, acute tolerance develops in subjects during an experiment as a function of administration schedules, and this tolerance influences the subjects' responses. Every attempt must be made to assess tolerance as it is induced. Adesso (1980) reminds us that tolerance is not a unitary phenomenon but an integrated process of many response systems that differentially adapt to alcohol. Researchers must therefore specify which dimensions of tolerance were assessed as well as which measures of tolerance were used.

Pre-Experimental Abstinence. In the studies that we surveyed, researchers have reported pre-experimental abstinence in subjects for periods ranging between one week (Vanderpool, 1969) and two months (McGuire and others, 1966). When subjects are recruited from correctional or treatment facilities, such variability in pre-experimental abstinence is unavoidable. In situations where researchers have a choice, however, Marlatt's (1978) abstinence violation effect (AVE) makes a period of pre-experimental abstinence seem unwise. The AVE predicts feelings of guilt and failure in relapsed alcoholics (in this case, relapsed through experimenter instruction), followed by a realignment of the self-concept to predispose the drinker to further negative effects. Thus, measurement of relapsed alcoholics' personalities may reflect the negative consequences of their having violated their vow to remain abstinent.

Subject Expectancies. It is well established that responses to alcohol are due both to learned expectancies about the effects of alcohol and to the actual pharmacological properties of alcohol. Thus, to clarify the role of alcohol in producing a certain effect, control of the intervening cognitive variable, expectancy, must be demonstrated.

An early method for controlling expectancy by keeping subjects naive as to their actual degree of intoxication replaced oral ingestion with intravenous alcohol infusion. This method, most notably used by Mayfield (1968a, 1968b), has been criticized both for its reactivity and for its lack of resemblance to the usual drinking setting. Its control of expectancy can fail, too, since some alcohol is expelled from the lungs, and sensitive subjects can detect its presence through smell and taste.

Another method of controlling expectancy, made popular by Marlatt and others (1973), is the balanced placebo design, a 2 × 2 factorial design. Half of the subjects in such an experiment are told to expect a dose of alcohol, while the other subjects are told to expect no alcohol. Actual beverages are carefully disguised, and half of each expectancy condition actually receives alcohol, while the other half receives no alcohol. With this design, it is possible to assess the relative contributions of expectancy effects and physiological effects to the overall effects of beverage consumption. Marlatt and Rohsenow (1980) discuss findings with the balanced placebo design in detail. However, like the alcohol infusion method, the balanced placebo design is not without problems. Such an experiment is expensive to conduct, since it requires four times the number of subjects tested in most chronic studies. Also, keeping subjects ignorant of the alcoholic content of their drinks over multiple drinking sessions is difficult, and there is some evidence that the deception fails at doses (or expected doses) above 50 mg/%. For this reason, a validity check—an assessment of the degree to which the subjects have accepted the experimenter's statement about the alcoholic content of their drinks—should always be conducted.

Despite these procedural difficulties, control of expectancy effects has yielded striking results. Wilson's work on sexual arousal, Mayfield's finding (which contradicts the results of most other researchers) that drinking can have positive affective sequelae for alcoholics, Marlatt's work on craving, and the contributions of others argue for the continued control of expectancy, although the infusion method and the balanced placebo design may not be the best procedures for meeting this requirement.

Subject Selection. The generalizability of studies of the effects of alcohol on alcoholics is limited by the dominance of skid row alcoholics as experimental subjects—subjects who are unrepresentative of the general alcoholic population on numerous critical variables. Only one study of the effects of alcohol on female alcoholics (Tracey and Nathan, 1976) has been conducted, and the consequences of drinking that it found differed markedly from those indicated by studies of males. Furthermore, an age bias in alcohol research is more than evident. Only one researcher (Williams, 1966) has examined the effects of alcohol on problem drinkers below the age of about thirty, and we know literally nothing about the effects of alcohol on the elderly alcoholic. It is most disturbing that the fastest-growing subgroups of the alcoholic population—the young, the female, and the elderly—are also those on which only the dimmest light has been shed. Experimental subjects have almost exclusively been thirty- to sixty-year-old, low socioeconomic status, single, hospitalized or incarcerated males.

Experimental Settings. The experimental settings of alcohol research are often artificial in the sense that they lack the social interactions that are characteristic of the real world and in the sense that both the mode (intravenous infusion) and the schedule (operant, programmed) of alcohol administration are often contrived. We should remember that the frequently cited findings of Mendelson and others (1964) that cast doubt on the tension reduction hypothesis—that is, subjects became more, not less, anxious and depressed as the drinking experiment continued—were based on subjects who were restricted to a hospital's neurological ward for the duration of the study and given alcohol, like it or not, every four hours, including 2:00 and 6:00 A.M. It is important to note that, in this study and many others, subjects' incremental deterioration of mood as drinking continued was confounded with a third incremental variable, namely time spent in a difficult experimental milieu. Subjects, including alcoholic subjects, respond to social, environmental, and temporal stimuli as well as to pharmacological stimuli. Thus, it probably is no accident that the few experimenters who attempted to create a natural living and drinking environment for their subjects (Steinglass, 1979; Tracey and Nathan, 1976) have reported results that are discrepant with the main body of research findings.

Dependent Measurement. We have noted the significant problems raised for study design by sample integrity, within-sample variability, assessment of BAL, tolerance and expectancy effects, pre-experimental abstinence, subject selection biases, and artificial experimental settings, but no problem looms as large as the problems related to dependent measurement. One major difficulty is the lack of uniformity in dependent measures employed by different studies. Measures have ranged from informal interviews and casual staff observations in most chronic studies to formal psychiatric inventories in most acute and a few chronic studies. Interview and observational data are never accompanied by reliability estimates, and no attempts have been made to shield the data from experimenter and rating biases. Formal instruments, such as the Mood Adjective Check List (MACL), the Psychiatric Outpatient Mood Scale, and the Clyde Mood Scale, are vulnerable to at least five limitations: First, original validation and reliability samples were generally composed of college students and psychiatric outpatients, and the instruments may require reading and educational levels beyond those of most alcoholic subjects (Freed, 1978). Second, no instrument, except the Clyde Mood Scale, was designed to measure the affective consequences of drug ingestion, and that scale has been used by only one researcher, Mayfield. Third, scales themselves are never reliable; only responses to scales are reliable, and we know literally nothing of our scales' reliability when they are administered to intoxicated subjects. Fourth, the effect of multiple administrations of a scale—for example, the MACL was given thirty times to each subject in the study by Nathan and others (1970)—on later responses to that scale are unknown. Fifth, our measures may themselves influence moods, as indicated by recent data (Perlmuter and others, in press) documenting the iatrogenic, mood-inducing properties of one popular instrument, the Beck Depression Inventory.

One alternative—curiously omitted from our scaling procedures—is the technique of magnitude estimation of alcohol's effects on affect pioneered by Ekman and others (1963) in Sweden. These researchers give social drinkers various concentrations of beverage alcohol (33–100 mg/%) while taking breath alcohol measures and observational measures of the drinkers' behavior. The sole estimate of self-reported affective change is obtained via magnitude estimation: Subjects rate the intensity of the subjective stimulus (affect) just as they would rate the intensity of a psychophysical stimulus, such as sound or light. Estimates of the magnitude of numerous intensive dimensions (for example, talkative, elated, happy, hazy, tense, tired) are made by the subjects on a numerical scale at frequent intervals. These data are then compared with the subjects' BALs and the observational data. Ekman and others (1963) reported remarkable correspondence between BAL, observational data, and subjects' magnitude estimates of the various dimensions just named. In most cases, the functions for BAL and positive affects are virtually indistinguishable, while negative affects (for example, tense) show an inverse correspondence with the BAL curve. The adaptation of this measurement strategy to the study of the subjective effects of alcohol on alcoholics, we feel, has much promise, and it is long overdue.

Concluding Remarks

The difficulty and ambiguity of the psychological researcher's task is nowhere better exemplified than in the growing body of critical treatises on it. On the one hand, the complex nature of our task has sometimes been viewed with concern, with authorities citing the complexity of our work as stifling to the conduct of our business and as aversive to newly attracted cadres of talent. We disagree. That more questions are raised than answered is as much as a behavioral researcher can ever ask. On the other hand, some reviewers of work in alcohol studies have laid a heavy onus on researchers for being too simple-minded, maintaining that "a large part of the problem appears to derive from investigators often ignoring important variables and conducting their research in ways that make interpretation of their results difficult" (Maisto and others, 1978, p. 243). Again we disagree, at least with the tone of the remark. We have no doubt that, like other work, research on the addictions manifests so many apparent ills only as a function of the increasing methodological sophistication that we demand of it.

Finally, in alcohol research, as in every other field of psychological endeavor, "our goals must be to strive toward conducting the least fallible inquiry, to cautiously interpret our experiments in accord with their logical warrant, and to guard against the paralysis of complacency regarding the adequacy of current research methods" (Mahoney, 1978, p. 660). We agree.

References

Adesso, V. J. "Experimental Studies of Human Drinking Behavior." In H. Rigter and J. C. Crabbe, Jr. (Eds.), *Alcohol Tolerance and Dependence.* New York: Elsevier/North Holland Biomedical Press, 1980.

Berg, N. L. "Effects of Alcohol Intoxication of Self-Concept." *Quarterly Journal of Studies on Alcohol,* 1971, *32,* 442–453.

Billings, A., Kessler, M., Gomberg, C., and Weiner, S. "Marital Conflict Resolution of Alcoholic and Nonalcoholic Couples During Drinking and Nondrinking Sessions." *Journal of Studies on Alcohol,* 1979, *40,* 183–195.

Caddy, G. R. "Toward a Multivariate Analysis of Alcohol Abuse." In P. E. Nathan, G. A. Marlatt, and T. Løberg (Eds.), *Alcoholism: New Directions in Behavioral Research and Treatment.* New York: Plenum, 1978.

Carpenter, J. A., and Armenti, N. P. "Some Behavioral Effects of Alcohol on Man." In B. Kissin and H. Begleiter (Eds.), *The Biology of Alcoholism.* Vol. 2.: *Physiology and Behavior.* New York: Plenum, 1972.

Cohen, M., Liebson, I., and Faillace, L. "The Role of Reinforcement Contingencies in Chronic Alcoholism: An Experimental Analysis of One Case." *Behavior Research and Therapy,* 1971, *9,* 375–379.

Conger, J. J. "Reinforcement Theory and the Dynamics of Alcoholism." *Quarterly Journal of Studies on Alcohol,* 1956, *17,* 296–305.

Cutter, H., Key, J., Rothstein, R., and Jones, W. "Alcohol, Power, and Inhibition." *Quarterly Journal of Studies on Alcohol,* 1973, *34,* 381–389.

Davis, D. "Mood Changes in Alcoholic Subjects with Programmed and Free-Choice Experimental Drinking." In N. Mello and J. Mendelson (Eds.), *Recent Advances in Studies of Alcoholism: An Interdisciplinary Approach.* Washington, D.C.: U.S. Government Printing Office, 1971.

Diethelm, O., and Barr, R. "Psychotherapeutic Interviews and Alcohol Intoxication." *Quarterly Journal of Studies on Alcohol,* 1962, *23,* 243–251.

Ekman, G., Frankenhauser, M., Goldberg, L., Bjerver, K., Järpe, G., and Myrsten, A. "Effects of Alcohol Intake on Subjective and Objective Variables Over a Five-Hour Period." *Psychopharmacologia,* 1963, *4,* 28–38.

Freed, E. X. "Alcohol and Mood: An Updated Review." *International Journal of the Addictions,* 1978, *13,* 173–200.

Funderbunk, F., and Allen, R. "Assessing the Alcoholic's Disposition to Drink." In M. M. Gross (Ed.), *Alcohol Intoxication and Withdrawal.* IIIB: *Studies in Alcohol Dependence.* New York: Plenum, 1977.

Glatt, M. M. "The Question of Moderate Drinking Despite 'Loss of Control.'" *British Journal of Addiction,* 1967, *62,* 267–274.

Gross, M., Rosenblatt, S., Lewis, E., Malenowski, B., and Broman, M. "Hallucinations and Clouding of Sensorium in Alcohol Withdrawal: Some Demographic and Cultural Relationships." *Quarterly Journal of Studies on Alcohol,* 1971, *32,* 1061–1069.

Hodgson, R., Rankin, H., and Stockwell, T. "Alcohol Dependence and the Priming Effect." *Behavior Research and Therapy,* 1979, *17,* 379–388.

Jellinek, E. M. *The Disease Concept of Alcoholism.* New Brunswick, N.J.: Hillhouse Press, 1960.

Johnson, L., Burdick, J., and Smith, J. "Sleep During Alcohol Intake and Withdrawal in the Chronic Alcoholic." *Archives of General Psychiatry,* 1970, *22,* 406–418.

Key, J., Cutter, H., Rothstein, R., and Jones, W. "Alcohol, Power, and Inhibition: A Factor Analytic Evaluation of McClelland's Hypothesis with a Construct Validation of the Factors." *Journal of Health and Social Behavior,* 1972, *13,* 337–346.

Ludwig, A., Wikler, A., and Stark, L. "The First Drink: The Psychological Aspects of Craving." *Archives of General Psychiatry,* 1974, *30,* 539–547.

Mahoney, M. J. "Experimental Methods and Outcome Research." *Journal of Consulting and Clinical Psychology,* 1978, *46,* 660–672.

Maisto, S., Connors, G., and Vuchinich, R. "Methodological Considerations in Alcohol Research with Human Subjects." *Addictive Behaviors,* 1978, *3,* 243–251.

Marlatt, G. A. "Craving for Alcohol, Loss of Control, and Relapse: A Cognitive-Behavioral Analysis." In P. E. Nathan, G. A. Marlatt, and T. Løberg (Eds.), *Alcoholism: New Directions in Behavioral Research and Treatment.* New York: Plenum, 1978.

Marlatt, G., Demming, B., and Reid, J. "Loss of Control Drinking in Alcoholics: An Experimental Analogue." *Journal of Abnormal Psychology,* 1973, *81,* 233–241.

Marlatt, G., and Rohsenow, D. "Cognitive Processes in Alcohol Use: Expectancy and the Balanced Plecebo Design." In N. K. Mello (Ed.), *Advances in Substance Abuse: Behavioral and Biological Research.* Greenwich, Conn.: JAI Press, 1980.

Matthews, D., and Miller, W. "Estimating Blood Alcohol Concentration: Two Computer Programs and Their Applications in Therapy and Research." *Addictive Behaviors,* 1979, *4,* 55–60.

Mayfield, D. G. "Psychopharmacology of Alcohol. I. Affective Change with Intoxication: Drinking Behavior and Affective State." *Journal of Nervous and Mental Disease,* 1968a, *146,* 314–321.

Mayfield, D. G. "Psychopharmacology of Alcohol. II. Affective Tolerance in Alcohol Intoxication." *Journal of Nervous and Mental Disease,* 1968b, *146,* 322–327.

Mayfield, D., and Allen, D. "Alcohol and Affect: A Psychopharmacological Study." *American Journal of Psychiatry,* 1967, *123,* 1345–1351.

McClelland, D., Davis, W., Kalin, R., and Wanner, W. *The Drinking Man.* New York: Free Press, 1972.

McGuire, M., Stein, S., and Mendelson, J. "Comparative Psychosocial Studies of Alcoholic and Nonalcoholic Subjects Undergoing Experimentally Induced Ethanol Intoxication." *Psychosomatic Medicine,* 1966, *28,* 13–26.

McNamee, H., Mello, N., and Mendelson, J. "Experimental Analysis of Drinking Patterns of Alcoholics: Concurrent Psychiatric Observations." *American Journal of Psychiatry,* 1968, *124,* 1063–1069.

Mello, N. K. "A Semantic Aspect of Alcoholism." In H. D. Cappell and A. E. LeBlanc (Eds.), *Biological and Behavioral Approaches to Drug Dependence.* Toronto: Addiction Research Foundation, 1975.

Mello, N., McNamee, H., and Mendelson, J. "Drinking Patterns of Chronic Alcoholics: Gambling and Motivation for Alcohol." In J. O. Cole (Ed.), *Clinical Research in Alcoholism.* Washington, D.C.: American Psychiatric Association, 1968.

Mello, N., and Mendelson, J. "A Quantitative Analysis of Drinking Patterns in Alcoholics." *Archives of General Psychiatry,* 1971, *27,* 527–539.

Menaker, T. "Anxiety and Drinking in Alcoholics." *Journal of Abnormal Psychology,* 1967, *72,* 43–49.

Mendelson, J., LaDou, J., and Solomon, P. "Experimentally Induced Chronic Intoxication and Withdrawal in Alcoholics. Part III: Psychiatric Findings." *Quarterly Journal of Studies on Alcohol,* 1964, Supplement No. 2, 40–52.

Mendelson, J., and Mello, N. "Experimental Analysis of Drinking Behavior of Chronic Alcoholics." *Annals of the New York Academy of Sciences,* 1966, *133,* 828–845.

Miller, W. R. "Alcoholism Scales and Objective Assessment Methods: A Review." *Psychological Bulletin,* 1976, *83,* 649–674.

Mueller, S. R. "The Effects of Alcohol upon the Alcoholic's Conformity Behavior and Mood State." Unpublished doctoral dissertation, Boston University, 1965.

Nathan, P., and O'Brien, J. "An Experimental Analysis of the Behavior of Alcoholics and Nonalcoholics During Prolonged Experimental Drinking: A Necessary Precursor of Behavior Therapy?" *Behavior Therapy,* 1971, *2,* 455–476.

Nathan, P., Titler, N., Lowenstein, L., Solomon, P., and Rossi, A. "Behavioral Analysis of Chronic Alcoholism." *Archives of General Psychiatry,* 1970, *22,* 419-430.

Nathan, P., Wilson, G., and Hay, W. Unpublished data. New Brunswick, N.J.: Alcohol Behavior Research Laboratory, Rutgers University, 1980.

Pattison, E. M. "Nonabstinent Drinking Goals in the Treatment of Alcoholism." In R. J. Gibbins and others (Eds.), *Research Advances in Alcohol and Drug Problems.* Vol. 3. New York: Wiley, 1976.

Pattison, E., Sobell, M., and Sobell, L. (Eds.). *Emerging Concepts of Alcohol Dependence.* New York: Springer, 1977.

Perlmuter, L., Noblin, C., and Hakami, M. "Reactive Effects of Tests for Depression: Theoretical and Methodological Considerations." *Journal of Social and Clinical Psychology,* in press.

Pihl, R., and Spiers, P. "Individual Characteristics in the Etiology of Drug Abuse." *Progress in Experimental Personality Research,* 1978, *8,* 93-195.

Sarason, I. G. *Personality: An Objective Approach.* New York: Wiley, 1966.

Skinner, H. A. "Assessment of Alcohol Problems: Basic Principles, Critical Issues, and Future Trends," In Y. Israel and others (Eds.), *Research Advances in Alcohol and Drug Problems.* Vol. 6. New York: Plenum, 1981.

Steinglass, P. "An Experimental Treatment Program for Alcoholic Couples." *Journal of Studies on Alcohol,* 1979, *40,* 159-182.

Tamerin, J., and Mendelson, J. "The Psychodynamics of Chronic Inebriation: Observation of Alcoholics During the Process of Drinking in an Experimental Group Setting." *American Journal of Psychiatry,* 1969, *125,* 886-899.

Tamerin, J., Weiner, S., and Mendelson, J. "Alcoholics' Expectancies and Recall of Experiences During Drinking." *American Journal of Psychiatry,* 1970, *126,* 1697-1704.

Tracey, D., and Nathan, P. "Behavioral Analysis of Chronic Alcoholism in Four Women." *Journal of Consulting and Clinical Psychology,* 1976, *44,* 832-842.

Vanderpool, J. A. "Alcoholism and Self-Concept." *Quarterly Journal of Studies on Alcohol,* 1969, *30,* 59-77.

van der Spuy, H. "The Influence of Alcohol on the Mood of the Alcoholic." *British Journal of Addiction,* 1972, *67,* 255-265.

Vannicelli, M. L. "Mood and Self-Perception of Alcoholics When Sober and Intoxicated. I. Mood Change. II. Accuracy of Self-Prediction." *Quarterly Journal of Studies on Alcohol,* 1972, *33,* 341-357.

Williams, A. F. "Social Drinking, Anxiety, and Depression." *Journal of Personality and Social Psychology,* 1966, *3,* 689-693.

Wilson, G., and Lawson, D. "Expectancies, Alcohol, and Sexual Arousal in Male Social Drinkers." *Journal of Abnormal Psychology,* 1976, *85,* 587-594.

Wilson, G., Lawson, D., and Abrams, D. "The Effects of Alcohol on Sexual Arousal in Male Alcoholics." *Journal of Abnormal Psychology,* 1978, *87,* 609-616.

Wolin, S., and Mello, N. "The Effects of Alcohol on Dreams and Hallucinations in Alcohol Addicts." *Annals of the New York Academy of Sciences,* 1973, *215,* 266-302.

James Langenbucher is a research assistant at the Alcohol Behavior Research Laboratory of Rutgers University and a doctoral student in clinical psychology at Rutgers University.

Peter E. Nathan is principal investigator of the Alcohol Behavior Research Laboratory, chair of the Department of Clinical Psychology, and director of clinical training at the Graduate School of Applied and Professional Psychology, Rutgers University.

Do alcoholics have an overly strong or an overly weak perception of their ability to control events that affect their lives? How does this perception affect treatment?

Alcoholics' Perceptions of Control

Damaris J. Rohsenow

Any professional who works with alcoholics soon becomes aware of the conflicts that surround the issue of control in the alcoholic's life. Clearly, alcoholics have lost control over their drinking. Usually, they also have failed to manage other areas of their lives, such as marriage and job. However, many alcoholics have an unrealistically strong belief in their ability to control their drinking, in spite of their repeated failures to do so. One of the principal aims of psychotherapy is to help people to gain more control over their lives. However, if it is true that alcoholics' perceptions of control are unwarrantedly strong, it may be beneficial to lessen their sense of control over events. Such issues as these led to research on alcoholics' locus on control and its relationship to treatment in hopes that the results would help to improve treatment approaches.

The concept of locus of control was developed within social learning theory by Rotter (1966) to refer to the degree to which a person generally perceives events as contingent on his or her own behavior or characteristics. Social learning theory deals in part with the effect of people's expectancies about events on their behavior. People with an internal locus of control generally believe that their behavior influences events, so they are more likely to make an effort to effect changes in themselves or in the world around them. People with an external locus of control tend to believe that events are a result of fate, chance, or powerful others. Therefore, they are not likely to perceive their own effect on events or to attempt to change them. This generalized notion of expectancy has been popular among researchers during the last fifteen years.

W. M. Cox (Ed.). *Identifying and Measuring Alcoholic Personality Characteristics.* New Directions for Methodology of Social and Behavioral Science, no. 16. San Francisco: Jossey-Bass, June 1983.

Locus of Control Scales

Most locus of control research with alcoholics has used one or another of six scales. The most widely used scale is Rotter's (1966) I-E scale, a twenty-three-item forced-choice scale scored in the external direction. It has good reliability and fairly good validity. Mirels (1970) found it useful to distinguish two factors of Rotter's I-E scale when studying alcoholics, since personality or treatment variables are often related to Personal Control but not to Sociopolitical Control. Whereas Rotter's scale measures an individual's perception of control over external events, the Experienced Control (EC) Scale developed by Tiffany and his associates (Tiffany, 1967; Tiffany and others, 1969) taps the individual's experience of four different kinds of control: experiencing control over internal organismic forces, feeling controlled by these forces, experiencing control over interpersonal or environmental forces, and feeling controlled by these forces. Two other scales have been used less frequently with alcoholics, but they have some advantages. The adult form of the Nowicki-Strickland scale (ANSIE, Nowicki and Duke, 1974) has a fifth-grade reading difficulty. A scale devised by Levenson (1973), which factor analytic and validity studies have supported, differentiates among three dimensions: internal control, control by powerful others, and control by chance.

Two newer scales show the most promise for research with alcoholics. Both have been designed specifically to assess the locus of control of drinking behavior. The Drinking-Related Locus of Control (DRIE) Scale (Keyson and Janda, 1972) measures expectancies of control over a variety of drinking-related behaviors. It has three factors: Intrapersonal Control—the degree to which a person resists the temptation to drink and drinks to change unpleasant moods; Interpersonal Control—the degree to which a person resists social pressure to drink and handles interpersonal anger; and General Control—chance factors influencing the individual's ability to stay sober (Donovan and O'Leary, 1978). Stafford's new Locus of Drinking Control (LODC) Scale (Stafford, 1980) is designed to assess perception of control over and responsibility for alcohol intake, intoxicated behavior, negative consequences of drinking, and etiology of the drinking problem. Relatively few studies have used these two scales.

Alcoholics Versus Nonalcoholics

Hypotheses. Three principal hypotheses have been proposed about differences in the locus of control for alcoholics and for nonalcoholics. The first hypothesis is that alcoholics have more external locus of control than nonalcoholics do, since alcoholics are unable to control both their drinking and other areas of their lives. The second hypothesis is that alcoholics have an unrealistically strong sense of control, since they often believe that they can control their drinking in spite of consistent failure to do so. The third hypothesis is that alcoholics have an internal locus of control that is realistic, since they have access to a substance that can increase pleasure and counteract unpleasant moods at any time.

Initially, it was expected that the first hypothesis would be supported, since internal locus of control has generally been associated with good psychosocial functioning. However, the initial studies found either that alcoholics scored more internally than controls did or that there was no significant difference between alcoholics and controls. Hence, the other two hypotheses were developed. Nevertheless, inspection revealed methodological problems in the early studies that rendered their conclusions invalid. Rohsenow and O'Leary, 1978a, provide details.

Methodological Problems. The first methodological problem was that I-E scores for alcoholic and control groups overlapped considerably across studies, so that alcoholics called *internal* in one study were labelled *external* in another. Second, the definition of *alcoholic* has not been consistent, and alcoholic samples have varied widely in severity and pattern of drinking problems as well as in demographic characteristics. These differences could correlate with locus of control. Third and most important, inappropriate nonalcoholic comparison samples have been used. Studies that found alcoholics to be significantly more internal than nonalcoholics compared middle-aged blue-collar workers who had roughly a twelfth-grade education with Rotter's (1966) college student norms, emotionally disturbed inpatients, inpatient opiate addicts, recovered alcoholic alcoholism counselors, or members of a church group. In all these cases, one can hardly conclude that alcoholism was the only difference between the alcoholic and control groups. Age, educational level, and psychosocial maladjustment have all been found to correlate with locus of control.

One other methodological problem needs to be considered. Virtually all the studies tested alcoholics in treatment. However, an alcoholic does not enter treatment unless the threatened unpleasant consequences of drinking, such as jail, divorce, or job loss, have become so strong and immediate that they outweigh the advantages. For this reason, alcoholics who undertake treatment are usually depressed about uncontrollable aversive events, and this temporary depression can result in increased externality. Alcoholics who do not seek treatment may well have a more internal perception of control.

Results of Better-Controlled Studies. Recent studies have used more appropriate comparison groups than early studies. For example, Butts and Chotlos (1973) used a control sample of the same age, educational level, and occupation as their alcoholic sample and found that the alcoholics were significantly more external on Rotter's scale. Donovan and O'Leary (1975) carefully matched alcoholics in Veterans Administration (VA) medical centers for age and educational level with nonalcoholic VA patients and employees and found no difference between the two groups on Rotter's I-E scale. However, they did find that the alcoholics experienced less control over interpersonal and intrapersonal pressures on the EC scale. Caster and Parsons (1977b) found that alcoholics scored higher on Levenson's scale than nonalcoholic middle-aged veterans in their belief about being controlled by chance events. In contrast, Donovan and others (1977) initially found no differences between alcoholics and matched nonalcoholics on Rotter's scale. However, after depression scores were covaried, the alcoholics became significantly more internal in locus of control than the nonalcoholics. Nevertheless, the alcoholics remained more external in their perceived control over drinking.

Other studies have found differences in locus of control within samples of nonalcoholic drinkers—that is, people whose drinking behavior does not warrant the diagnosis of alcoholism. For example, Naditch (1975) studied a large sample of army trainees and found that the more they drank, the more external their I-E scores became. Problem drinkers had the most external scores. Rohsenow (1982) found that heavy student drinkers were more external than light drinkers.

Two studies have looked at specific areas of control. These studies found that alcoholics felt significantly less in control of drinking-related behaviors on the Drinking-Related Locus of Control Scale than matched nonalcoholics (Donovan and O'Leary, 1978) and that female alcoholics perceived that they had less control over their sex life than matched nonalcoholics did (Pinhas, 1978).

In summary, virtually all the studies that use adequate control groups have found that alcoholics and problem drinkers are more external in locus of control than nonproblem drinkers are, both in general and specifically for drinking behaviors. Nevertheless, the possible confounding influences of depression and of being in treatment need to be clarified in future studies.

Self-Regulation. One study used measures other than locus of control scales to explore perceptions of control. Tarbox (1979) assessed actual and perceived self-control in alcoholics and matched nonalcoholics and found that the alcoholics had less impulse control and that they made more errors on a self-monitoring task than the nonalcoholics did, although the two groups did not differ in their average self-ratings of competence or in their predictions of their performance on cognitive and motor tasks. Furthermore, the alcoholics in this study overestimated their ability more often than the nonalcoholics did: The more errors they made, the more competent they believed themselves to be, in contrast to the nonalcoholics. This study supports the idea that alcoholics have an unrealistically strong belief in their own control over events, and it suggests that the perception of control over events alone may be less important than the discrepancy perceived and actual control.

Relationship to Other Personality Factors

Research with nonalcoholic groups has found that people with more external locus of control tend to be more anxious, aggressive, dogmatic, depressed, and suspicious and to be generally less well adjusted and less able to control themselves and their environment than people with more internal locus of control (Phares, 1976). Do these relationships hold for alcoholics as well? A review of the literature confirms that the patterns for alcoholics are generally consistent with the patterns for nonalcoholic populations. (See Rohsenow and O'Leary, 1978b, for details.) For example, many studies have found that externally scoring alcoholic males express more physical complaints, anxiety, depression, isolation, alienation, and general clinical pathology than internally scoring alcoholic males. Other studies have found that internal alcoholics use the more adaptive defenses, such as denial, intellectualization, and repression, while external alcoholics tend to turn against their perceived source of frustration as a defense mechanism. Two studies that administered an unobtrusive anxiety questionnaire found no differences in anxiety between internals and externals. This finding raises the possibility that the differences in anxiety that other studies have found reflect a difference in willingness to express self-critical descriptions more than they reflect actual differences in emotional state. However, since no consistent relationship has been found between locus of control and social desirability response bias (a measure of willingness to make self-critical statements), it is unlikely that this possible source of confounding poses a serious methodological problem.

The relationship of locus of control to interpersonal style has also been studied. Surprisingly, no relationship has been found between locus of control and either expressed or desired control on Shultz's FIRO-B scale of interpersonal relating. However, researchers have found that internal alcoholics express more need for social inclusion and affection and more assertiveness and less anger and aggression than external alcoholics do (Greenberg and others, 1978; Sturgis and others, 1979). However, despite the positive characteristics shown by internal alcoholics, hospital staff like helpless alcoholics significantly more (O'Leary and others, 1980). This is important because staff liking of patients has been found to be the primary determinant in decisions to continue treatment of alcoholics (O'Leary, Donovan, Chaney, and O'Leary, 1979).

A few variables seem to have no consistent relationship with locus of control among alcoholics. Studies correlating the age or intelligence of alcoholics with locus of control have had mixed results, while a number of studies have found that field dependence (a cognitive style) is unrelated to control orientation. In addition, investigators have not been able to identify any consistent sex differences in the locus of control of alcoholics. This is important because nearly all the studies that have compared the locus of control of alcoholics and nonalcoholics and that have investigated treatment effects on locus of control have studied only men. The absence of a sex difference suggests that the results of the studies of locus of control with men can be generalized to women.

The body of research has one significant shortcoming: The studies described here have used paper-and-pencil measures. Alcoholics' actual behavior has not been observed. However, there is evidence that paper-and-pencil measures correlate better with other paper-and-pencil measures than they do with actual behavior (Mischel, 1968). This does not necessarily imply that the relationships observed for alcoholics are invalid. It is true that we do not know what results would be obtained if we monitored the actual behavior of alcoholics.

In summary, internally scoring alcoholics tend to appear better adjusted than externals do on a variety of paper-and-pencil measures, as expected. Alcoholics who feel more helpless are better liked by hospital staff, perhaps because they are also more anxious and depressed and because they have less effective means of coping.

Relationship to Drinking-Related Problems

External locus of control has been found to be associated with reports of drinking-related physical, social, and emotional problems on the Alcohol Use Inventory (Wanberg and others, 1977). In one study (O'Leary and others, 1978), alcoholics who scored in the external direction on the EC scale also reported many maladaptive consequences of drinking and impaired physical and psychosocial functioning. In contrast, external scores on the I-E scale were found to have little relationship with drinking problems; instead, they correlated with drinking to enhance social abilities. The different outcomes with the two scales may result from the fact that the EC scale measures the experience of control over intrapersonal as well as environmental forces, while the I-E scale taps only the perception of control over external forces. The findings with the I-E scale are consistent with other data from heavy social drinkers: Externality on the I-E scale correlates highly with drinking to enhance social functioning ($r = .54$, $p < .001$, $N = 33$) but not with drinking problems and not with the actual alcohol consumed during the six months following testing (Rohsenow, 1982a). However, alcoholics who report less control over drinking behaviors on the DRIE Scale also report significantly more alcohol-related problems (Donovan and O'Leary, 1978). Since the Alcohol Use Inventory shows good predictive validity with alcoholics (Wanberg and others, 1977) and with heavy social drinkers (Rohsenow, 1982b), the results described here raise no particular methodological problems, although the observed correlations could be an artifact of the willingness of externally scoring individuals to report their weaknesses.

Finally, researchers have found a correlation between external locus of control on Rotter's scale and on the two drinking control scales and number of times in treatment (Oziel and Obitz, 1975; Rose and others, 1978; Stafford, 1980). Thus, alcoholics who perceive themselves as having little control may have great difficulty in learning to cope with their alcoholism.

In summary, it appears that alcoholics who report that they have little control over intrapersonal and environmental forces and over their own drinking also report severe problems from drinking and numerous unsuccessful treatment attempts. Conversely, alcoholics who only report feeling little control over external events are likely to report using alcohol to improve their social functioning and to have had numerous treatment attempts but not to report adverse consequences of drinking.

Treatment and Locus of Control

As already indicated, clinical researchers have assumed that it would be desirable for alcoholics to increase their sense of control, since internal locus of control has been associated with increased responsibility for actions, decisions, and their consequences and with active coping with the environment (Phares, 1976). Accordingly, researchers have hypothesized that alcoholics would increase their sense of internal locus of control during treatment and that this development would be associated with success in treatment. They have also hypothesized that external alcoholics would prefer to rely on structured supports in treatment, while internal alcoholics would prefer treatment emphasizing development of self-control. This section reviews findings related to these two hypotheses.

Treatment Choice by Alcoholics. Consistent with the prediction that patients with an external locus of control would prefer more structure and more external supports, Obitz (1978) found that alcoholics who chose to take disulfiram during treatment were more external than alcoholics who did not request disulfiram. Similarly, Stafford (1980) found that alcoholics who reported less control over their drinking-related behaviors were more likely to report wanting help in dealing with the alcohol problem than to refuse it and that they were more likely to accept a disease model than a sociopsychological model of alcoholism. However, Pachman and others (1978) found no relation between control orientation and choice of abstinence or a controlled drinking treatment as the goal.

Change in Control Orientation During Treatment. Although three studies (Burtle and others, 1974; Caster and Parsons, 1977a; Costello and Manders, 1974) found no change in alcoholics' locus of control during treatment, four other studies found that alcoholics increased their perceptions of control over the course of treatment as measured by the I-E, EC, and DRIE scales (Chess and others, 1971; O'Leary and others, 1975; Donovan and O'Leary, 1975; Obitz and Oziel, 1978). In fact, the longer that alcoholics participated in treatment, the more internal their locus of control became (Walker and others, 1979). Studies investigating whether alcoholics with internal or external initial scores are more likely to become more internal during treatment have found inconsistent results. One study (Greenberg and others, 1978) found that only external alcoholics became more internal in perceived control. Another study (Donovan and O'Leary, 1975) found that only internals became more internal in experienced control. Still another study (unpublished data from O'Leary, Rohsenow, and Chaney, 1979) found that both internals and externals became significantly more internal in perceived control during treatment. Thus, we cannot reach a definite conclusion about the effect that initial locus of control scores have on changes in perceived control during treatment.

One methodological difficulty encountered in interpretation of changes in control orientation during treatment is raised by the fact that initial scores are confounded with the life situation of the alcoholic at the time when he or she enters treatment. As already indicated, alcoholics often enter treatment at a time when they are extremely unhappy about the unpleasant or threatened consequences of their drinking. This means that their locus of control scores can reflect a relatively temporary state resulting from recent aversive events in their lives, not a typical sense of being out of control. Entering a treatment program can relieve many of the negative social and physical consequences of drinking, thereby alleviating the immediate crisis and effecting a return to a sense of being in control (Smith, 1970). Hence, it is possible that an enduring trait is not being changed during treatment but rather that a temporary and uncharacteristic state of feeling not in control of events is decreased by the passage of time and by escape from unpleasant pressures, which allows the individual to return to the usual sense of control. However, the existing research is unable to clarify this possibility.

In summary, the evidence appears to support the expectation that alcoholics gain an increased sense of control over their lives and drinking problems during treatment. However, it is not entirely clear whether the change is in a stable personality trait or whether it is a temporary change due to environmental conditions.

Locus of Control and Treatment Attrition. Attrition from treatment is generally considered to be a indirect indication of treatment failure, and it is important to determine whether attrition is related to alcoholics' perception of control. One study (Schofield, 1978) found that the scores of alcoholics who dropped out of an Alcoholics Anonymous–oriented program were more external than the scores of alcoholics who remained in treatment. Another study (Bowen and Twemlow, 1978) found no relationship between locus of control and attrition from a six-week Veterans Administration program. However, this result may be due to the short time period investigated, since three other studies from a different VA population found that, although there was no relation between locus of control and attrition from the five- to eight-week inpatient phase, locus of control was related to attrition from the nine months of weekly aftercare following the inpatient phase. O'Leary and others (1976) found that patients with more internal scores at the end of the inpatient treatment were more likely to drop out during the nine months of aftercare. In contrast, O'Leary and others (1977) and O'Leary, Rohsenow, and Chaney (1979) found that, after the effect of depression was covaried from the initial scores, patients with more internal locus of control were more likely to drop out of the aftercare program. These results are contrary to predicted outcomes. One possible explanation for them is that patients with external scores need to feel dependent on the structure of an aftercare program, while patients with internal scores believe that they can cope without additional treatment.

Interpretation of the results on attrition from treatment is not clear-cut. Although treatment attrition is usually assumed to indicate treatment failure, it would seem possible instead that patients who drop out do so because they are better able to cope effectively with their drinking problems at that point than other patients are. However, when we consider the fact that alcoholics who do return to excessive drinking after treatment are less likely than others to continue with their aftercare program, it seems plausible that aftercare attrition does in fact provide a rough index of failure.

In summary, contrary to prediction, treatment attrition occurs more often among internal alcoholics than it does among external alcoholics. This difference may reflect the reliance of external alcoholics on external supports, or it may reflect either a realistic or an unrealistic perception of control on the part of internal alcoholics.

Locus of Control and Treatment Outcome. Treatment outcome has been investigated by assessing the amount of drinking at follow-up. Rather than asking whether the patient is drinking or not and assuming that drinking reflects treatment failure, these studies have usually assessed the amount of drinking and classified the considerably improved drinkers and the abstainers as treatment successes and the drinkers who show no improvement or only slight improvement as treatment failures. Nevertheless, one difficulty with treatment outcome studies is that many alcoholics cannot be found at follow-up. To prevent outcome data from showing an inflated success rate, the missing alcoholics must be counted as treatment failures (Nathan and Lansky, 1978). For example, if 70 percent of the patients who start treatment are missing at follow-up it is inappropriate to claim an 80 percent success rate based on the patients who can be located. It is also important for the follow-up period to be long enough to reveal the lasting effects of treatment. A period of at least twelve months and as long as twenty-four months between termination of treatment and follow-up evaluation is usually recommended (Nathan and Lansky, 1978).

Most studies have found a relation between internal locus of control and improvement in drinking rate at follow-up. For instance, Caster and Parsons (1977a) found that treatment failures from an outpatient program utilizing behavior therapy and disulfiram had a greater belief in the role of chance in their lives (as indicated by Levenson's scale) than treatment successes did. Similarly, a behavior therapy program for female alcoholics in Germany that had abstinence as its treatment goal found that alcoholics who became controlled drinkers had a more internal locus of control at the end of treatment than either abstainers or treatment failures (Appelt, 1979). The hypothesis that alcoholics benefit most from treatment that stresses a control style that is congruent with their locus of control was not supported in a study by Schmidt

(1978): Internals fared better than externals whether treatment stressed self-control or reliance on a therapy group. Several other studies have found no significant relationship between locus of control and treatment outcome: Caster and Parsons (1977b) found no relationship between locus of control scores from Levenson's scale and treatment outcome for alcoholics in an in-patient insight-oriented program, and Miller and Joyce (1979) found that, when data were combined from four different behavioral studies, I-E scores were unrelated to treatment outcome. Only one study (Chaney, 1976) found results opposite to prediction: In an inpatient Veterans Administration program that stressed the development of responsibility, alcoholics who were more external at the start of treatment engaged in significantly less drinking and were significantly less often drunk during the year following treatment than internal alcoholics were.

The drinking outcomes in the studies just mentioned are based on alcoholics' own self-reports. The validity of such self-reports naturally falls into question. However, in recent years, the accuracy of self-reported drinking data from alcoholics has been checked against the reports of collateral informants—friends or family members—and legal and hospital records. Since the self-reports have been found to be quite reliable and valid (Sobell, 1978; Miller and others, 1979), we have little reason to question the accuracy of outcome data from the studies just reviewed.

In summary, the majority of treatment outcome studies have found that even though the individual's belief in his or her ability to exert control over events is associated with a tendency to drop out of extended aftercare treatment, patients who have this belief also have fewer drinking-related problems following treatment and greater treatment success in general. There are some discrepancies in the results of individual studies, but the discrepancies may result either from variations in treatment techniques among the various programs or from sample differences. One of the most important unanswered questions in treatment outcome research is whether internals and externals respond differentially to different treatment approaches. In other areas of psychotherapy research, internals have been found to respond favorably to non-directive approaches and to approaches focusing on control by the client, while externals have been found to respond well to structured approaches (Strickland, 1978). In the studies reviewed here between internal and external alcoholics, the differences in treatment do not appear to be related to program orientation, whether it was behavioral or disease-oriented (the Alcoholics Anonymous model). Nevertheless, the question of whether internals and externals respond differently to different treatment approaches has not been thoroughly investigated. Also, the relationship between drinking-related locus of control and treatment outcome has not been investigated, although drinking-related control could prove to be an important predictor of alcoholics' response to treatment.

Implications and Future Directions

What do these results mean for clinicians who work with alcoholics? It appears that alcoholics who feel least in control are at high risk for becoming treatment failures. Treatment staff could take advantage of these alcoholics' greater need to be dependent on external supports by encouraging them, for example, to use disulfiram and to join an aftercare group that could help them to cope with difficulties. Alternatively, treatment could focus on developing the belief of these alcoholics that their own behavior can have an effect on their environment, so that they will be less likely to allow external events and peer pressure to control their behavior. Cognitive therapy techniques (Beck and others, 1979) could be adapted to teach patients to recognize the effects that their own behavior can have. Social skills training could also be used to this end—by increasing alcoholics' actual ability to modify both their environment and their moods and by providing them with feedback from peers that demonstrates how their role-played interactions affect others. One study that used the latter approach found particularly effective results for alcoholics with an external locus of control. (See Chaney and others, 1978, for details of the treatment.) Alcoholics who believe that they have the ability to control their own life may not be liked by treatment staff, because this belief is contrary to traditional treatment philosophies. Although such alcoholics are more likely to drop out of an aftercare program, they are also more likely to be successful in the long run than external alcoholics are if they stay in the initial treatment program. Accordingly, the best approach for these alcoholics may be to ensure that their abilities correspond to their beliefs by teaching them effective methods for coping with situations that commonly lead to relapse. Marlatt and Gordon (1979) provide some useful suggestions.

What methodological details does future research need to consider? First, potentially confounding variables must be controlled by careful matching of alcoholic groups with nonalcoholic comparison groups. Because this requirement has not been met in past research, our information about alcoholics' locus of control comes from alcoholics who are undergoing treatment, and it is impossible to know whether the observed perceptions of control are a consequence of the patients' alcoholism or of the events that led them to seek treatment. Accordingly, we need data from alcoholics who are not undergoing treatment. Second, most studies have used global questionnaire measures of psychosocial functioning. However, it would be useful to have more objective measures of the actual functioning of alcoholics. Behavioral observations or official records could be used to obtain such measures. Third, one useful change that has already occurred involves a shift from assessment of global control orientation to more specific expectancies of control. Development of drinking-related locus of control scales, for instance, is likely to prove extremely productive. Alcoholics' perceptions of control over politics, jobs, and school performance are less likely to be relevant predictors of their treatment success than perceptions of control over drinking-related behaviors.

What fruitful directions can future research take? One interesting possibility is to study alcoholics' attributions about different aspects of their alcoholism. They may have different attributions for the causes of their alcoholism and for the success or failure of their treatment, but their attributions about the latter are more likely to have an impact on actual treatment outcomes. In this connection, a Drinking Attributional Style Scale (Rohsenow, 1981) is being developed to assess the stability, globality, and internality of attributions about six different aspects of drinking. Thus, the relationship of these attributions to treatment outcome can be studied in future research.

Another productive direction for future research involves the effects on actual drinking behavior of expectancies about the effects of alcohol. It is possible that people seek to lose control over some actions and drink to excuse irresponsible behavior. A series of studies on expectancy effects (Marlatt and Rohsenow, 1980) shows that the belief that alcohol has been consumed can result in loss of control and in craving among alcoholics as well as in changes in physical aggression, sexual arousal (especially to deviant scenes, such as rape), laughter, and social anxiety among social drinkers. However, the pharmacological effects of moderate doses of alcohol have no effect on these behaviors. Hence, alcohol may provide the ideal excuse for engaging in behaviors that normally are disapproved. Other people attribute the behavior to the alcohol, not to the drinker. If this goal of drinking is ignored, treatment efforts will be less effective for many alcoholics. Treatment approaches can perhaps be improved by assessing the areas in which alcoholics seek to lose control, then by providing training in other ways that allow them to attain their goals. Miller and Muñoz (1982) provide some suggestions.

Another promising area for future research on perceptions of control is alcoholics' self-efficacy expectancies—their estimates of their ability to cope successfully with troublesome situations (Bandura, 1977). Even if alcoholics receive considerable training in coping skills, they are not likely to use them successfully if they do not believe that they can cope effectively with a situation. The potential utility of this approach has been demonstrated in a treatment study with smokers (Condiotte and Lichtenstein, 1981) in which subjects rated the probability that they would be able to resist the urge to smoke in forty-eight situations that commonly lead to relapse for smokers. The situation that a smoker had the lowest confidence about handling was indeed the situation in which he or she relapsed. If we assessed the areas about which an alcoholic had the lowest self-efficacy expectations, then treatment could be tailored to meet the alcoholics' particular needs.

In conclusion, research on alcoholics' perceptions of control began with global personality measures, but increasingly it has moved toward assessing specific expectancies of control. These specific expectancies show considerable promise for improving treatment strategies within the next decade.

References

Appelt, H. "Depression and Locus of Control Among Female Alcoholics and Their Significance in Treatment Outcome." *Behavior Analysis and Modification,* 1979, *3,* 143–151.

Bandura, A. "Self-Efficacy: Toward a Unifying Theory of Behavioral Change." *Psychological Review,* 1977, *84,* 191–215.

Beck, A. T., Rush, A. J., Shaw, B. F., and Emergy, G. *Cognitive Therapy of Depression.* New York: Guilford Press, 1979.

Bowen, W. T., and Twemlow, S. W. "Locus of Control and Treatment Dropout in an Alcoholic Population." *British Journal of Addiction,* 1978, *73,* 51–54.

Burtle, V., Whitlock, D., and Franks, V. "Modification of Low Self-Esteem in Women Alcoholics: A Behavior Treatment Approach." *Psychotherapy: Research and Practice,* 1974, *11,* 36–40.

Butts, S. V., and Chotlos, J. "A Comparison of Alcoholics and Nonalcoholics on Perceived Locus of Control." *Quarterly Journal of Studies on Alcohol,* 1973, *34,* 1327–1332.

Caster, D. U., and Parsons, O. A. "Locus of Control in Alcoholics and Treatment Outcome." *Journal of Studies on Alcohol,* 1977a, *38,* 2087–2095.

Caster, D. U., and Parsons, O. A. "Relationship of Depression, Sociopathy, and Locus of Control to Treatment Outcome in Alcoholics." *Journal of Consulting and Clinical Psychology,* 1977b, *45,* 751–756.

Chaney, E. F. "Skill Training with Alcoholics." Unpublished doctoral dissertation, University of Washington, Seattle, 1976.

Chaney, E. F., O'Leary, M. R., and Marlatt, G. A. "Skill Training with Alcoholics." *Journal of Consulting and Clinical Psychology,* 1978, *46,* 1092–1104.

Chess, S. B., Neuringer, C., and Goldstein, G. "Arousal and Field Dependency in Alcoholics." *Journal of General Psychology,* 1971, *85,* 93–102.

Condiotte, M. M., and Lichtenstein, E. "Self-Efficacy and Relapse in Smoking Cessation Programs." *Journal of Consulting and Clinical Psychology,* 1981, *49,* 648–658.

Costello, R. M., and Manders, K. R. "Locus of Control and Alcoholism." *British Journal of Addiction,* 1974, *69,* 11–17.

Donovan, D. M., and O'Leary, M. R. "Comparison of Perceived and Experienced Control Among Alcoholics and Nonalcoholics." *Journal of Abnormal Psychology,* 1975, *84,* 726–728.

Donovan, D. M., and O'Leary, M. R. "The Drinking-Related Locus of Control Scale: Reliability, Factor Structure, and Validity." *Journal of Studies on Alcohol,* 1978, *39,* 759–784.

Donovan, D. M., Radford, L. M., Chaney, E. F., and O'Leary, M. R. "Perceived Locus of Control as a Function of Level of Depression Among Alcoholics and Nonalcoholics." *Journal of Clinical Psychology,* 1977, *33,* 582–584.

Greenberg, E. A., Obitz, F. W., and Kaye, B. W. "Relationships among Control Orientation, the FIRO-B, and the Ward Atmosphere Scale in Hospitalized Men Alcoholics." *Journal of Studies on Alcohol,* 1978, *39,* 68–76.

Keyson, M., and Janda, L. *The Drinking-Related Locus of Control Scale.* Phoenix, Ariz: Saint Lukes Hospital, 1972.

Levenson, H. "Reliability and Validity of the I, P, and C Scales: A Multi-dimensional View of Locus of Control." Paper presented at 81st annual convention of the American Psychological Association, Montreal, 1973.

Marlatt, G. A., and Gordon, J. R. "Determinants of Relapse: Implications for the Maintenance of Behavior Change." In P. O. Davidson and S. M. Davidson (Eds.), *Behavioral Medicine: Changing Health Lifestyles.* New York: Brunner/Mazel, 1980.

Marlatt, G. A., and Rohsenow, D. J. "Cognitive Processes in Alcohol Use: Expectancy and the Balanced Placebo Design." In N. K. Mello (Ed.), *Advances in Substance*

Abuse: Behavioral and Biological Research. Vol. 1. Greenwich, Conn.: JAI Press, 1980.

Miller, W. R., Crawford, V. L., and Taylor, C. A. "Significant Others as Corroborative Sources for Problem Drinkers." *Addictive Behaviors,* 1979, *4,* 67–70.

Miller, W. R., and Joyce, M. A. "Prediction of Abstinence, Controlled Drinking, and Heavy Drinking Outcomes Following Behavioral Self-Control Training." *Journal of Consulting and Clinical Psychology,* 1979, *47,* 773–775.

Miller, W. R., and Muñoz, R. F. *How to Control Your Drinking.* Englewood Cliffs, N.J.: Prentice-Hall, 1982.

Mirels, H. L. "Dimensions of Internal Versus External Control." *Journal of Consulting and Clinical Psychology,* 1970, *34,* 226–228.

Mischel, W. *Personality and Assessment.* New York: Wiley, 1968.

Naditch, M. P. "Locus of Control and Drinking Behavior in a Sample of Men in Army Basic Training." *Journal of Consulting and Clinical Psychology,* 1975, *43,* 96.

Nathan, P. E., and Lansky, D. "Common Methodological Problems in Research on the Addictions." *Journal of Consulting and Clinical Psychology,* 1978, *46,* 713–726.

Nowicki, S., Jr., and Duke, M. P. "A Locus of Control Scale for Noncollege as Well as College Adults." *Journal of Personality Assessment,* 1974, *38,* 136–137.

Obitz, F. W. "Control Orientation and Disulfiram." *Journal of Studies on Alcohol,* 1978, *39,* 1297–1298.

Obitz, F. W., and Oziel, L. J. "Change in General and Specific Perceived Locus of Control in Alcoholics as a Function of Treatment Exposure." *International Journal of the Addictions,* 1978, *13,* 995–1001.

O'Leary, M. R., Donovan, D. M., Chaney, E. F., and O'Leary, D. E. "Interpersonal Attractiveness and Clinical Decisions in Alcoholism Treatment." *American Journal of Psychiatry,* 1979, *136,* 618–622.

O'Leary, M. R., Donovan, D. M., Cysewski, B., and Chaney, E. F. "Perceived Locus of Control, Experienced Control, and Depression: A Trait Description of the Learned Helplessness Model of Depression." *Journal of Clinical Psychology,* 1977, *33,* 164–168.

O'Leary, M. R., Donovan, D. M., Hague, W. H., and Shea, R. A. "Shifts in Component Factors of Locus of Control as a Function of Treatment in Male Alcoholics." *Journal of Clinical Psychology,* 1975, *31,* 359–361.

O'Leary, M. R., Donovan, D. M., and O'Leary, D. E. "Drinking Patterns of Alcoholics Differing in Levels of Perceived and Experienced Control." *Journal of Studies on Alcohol,* 1978, *39,* 1499–1505.

O'Leary, M. R., Rohsenow, D. J., and Chaney, E. F. "The Use of Multivariate Personality Strategies in Predicting Attrition from Alcoholism Treatment." *Journal of Clinical Psychiatry,* 1979, *40,* 190–193.

O'Leary, M. R., Rohsenow, D. J., and Donovan, D. M. "Locus of Control and Patient Attrition from an Alcoholism Treatment Program." *Journal of Consulting and Clinical Psychology,* 1976, *44,* 686–687.

O'Leary, M. R., Speltz, M. L., and Walker, R. D. "Influence of Reported Helplessness on Client-Clinician Relationships in an Alcoholism Program." *Hospital and Community Psychiatry,* 1980, *31,* 783–784.

Oziel, L. J., and Obitz, F. W. "Control Orientation in Alcoholics Related to Extent of Treatment." *Journal of Studies on Alcohol,* 1975, *36,* 158–161.

Pachman, J. S., Foy, D. W., and Van-Erd, M. "Goal Choice of Alcoholics: A Comparison of Those Who Choose Total Abstinence Versus Those Who Choose Responsible Controlled Drinking." *Journal of Clinical Psychology,* 1978, *34,* 781–783.

Phares, E. J. *Locus of Control in Personality.* Morristown, N.J.: General Learning Press, 1976.

Pinhas, V. L. "An Investigation to Compare the Degree to Which Alcoholic and Nonalcoholic Women Report Sex Guilt and Sexual Control." Unpublished doctoral dissertation, New York University, 1978.

Rohsenow, D. J. *The Drinking Attributional Style Scale.* Unpublished scale, University of Wisconsin-Madison, 1981.

Rohsenow, D. J. "Social Anxiety, Daily Moods, and Alcohol Use over Time Among Heavy Social Drinking Men." *Addictive Behaviors,* 1982a, *7,* 311-315.

Rohsenow, D. J. "The Alcohol Use Inventory as Predictor of Drinking by Male Heavy Social Drinkers." *Addictive Behaviors,* 1982b, *7,* 387-395.

Rohsenow, D. J. "Control over Interpersonal Evaluation and Alcohol Consumption in Male Social Drinkers." *Addictive Behaviors,* 1982c, *7,* 113-121.

Rohsenow, D. J., and O'Leary, M. R. "Locus of Control Research on Alcoholic Populations: A Review. I. Development, Scales, and Treatment." *International Journal of the Addictions,* 1978a, *13,* 55-78.

Rohsenow, D. J., and O'Leary, M. R. "Locus of Control Research on Alcoholic Populations: A Review. II. Relationship to Other Measures." *International Journal of the Addictions,* 1978b, *13,* 213-226.

Rose, G. S., Powell, B. J., and Penick, E. C. "Determinants of Locus of Control Orientation in Male Alcoholics." *Journal of Clinical Psychology,* 1978, *34,* 250-251.

Rotter, J. B. "Generalized Expectancies for Internal Versus External Control of Reinforcement." *Psychological Monographs,* 1966, *80* (1), (entire issue).

Schmidt, M. R. "Structuring Treatment Programs on the Basis of Control Orientation of Alcoholics." Unpublished doctoral dissertation, University of Nebraska-Lincoln, 1978.

Schofield, L. J., Jr. "Internal-External Control and Withdrawal AMA from an Alcohol Rehabilitation Program." *Journal of Clinical Psychology,* 1978, *34,* 571-573.

Smith, R. E. "Changes in Locus of Control as a Function of Life Crisis Resolution." *Journal of Abnormal Psychology,* 1970, *75,* 328-332.

Sobell, L. C. "A Critique of Alcoholism Treatment Evaluation." In G. A. Marlatt and P. E. Nathan (Eds.), *Behavioral Approaches to Alcoholism.* New Brunswick, N.J.: Center of Alcohol Studies, Rutgers University, 1978.

Stafford, R. A. "Alcoholics' Perception of the Internal-External Locus of Their Drinking Problem." *Journal of Studies on Alcohol,* 1980, *41,* 300-309.

Strickland, B. R. "Internal-External Expectancies and Health-Related Behaviors." *Journal of Consulting and Clinical Psychology,* 1978, *46,* 1192-1211.

Sturgis, E. T., Calhoun, K. S., and Best, C. L. "Correlates of Assertive Behavior in Alcoholics." *Addictive Behaviors,* 1979, *4,* 193-197.

Tarbox, A. R. "Self-Regulation and Sense of Competence in Men Alcoholics." *Journal of Studies on Alcohol,* 1979, *40,* 860-866.

Tiffany, D. W. "Mental Health: A Function of Experienced Control." *Journal of Clinical Psychology,* 1967, *23,* 311-315.

Tiffany, D. W., Shontz, F. C., and Woll, S. B. "A Model of Control." *Journal of General Psychology,* 1969, *81,* 67-82.

Walker, R. D., Nast, E. C., Chaney, E. F., and O'Leary, M. R. "Changes in Drinking-Related Locus of Control as a Function of Length of Alcoholism Treatment." *Psychological Reports,* 1979, *44,* 287-293.

Wanberg, K. W., Horn, J. L., and Foster, F. M. "A Differential Assessment Model for Alcoholism: The Scales of the Alcohol Use Inventory." *Journal of Studies on Alcohol,* 1977, *38,* 512-543.

Damaris J. Rohsenow is assistant professor of clinical psychology at the University of Wisconsin-Madison.

Research of the past decade reveals differences between alcoholic men and women in a variety of personality characteristics and life experiences.

Gender Differences in Alcoholic Personality Characteristics and Life Experiences

Carole S. Benson
Sharon C. Wilsnack

Traditionally, alcoholism has been viewed as a predominantly male problem. Most early studies of alcoholism—for example, those attempting to identify an alcoholic personality (Cox, 1979)—did not include female alcoholics. Researchers seemed to assume that whatever was learned about alcoholism from men ought to apply equally well to women. Thus, although there are now an estimated two million problem drinking and alcoholic women in the United States, female drinkers received very little attention in the literature on alcohol problems until recently. In the absence of empirical data, much of what both lay and professional people believed they knew about female alcoholism and about male-female differences in alcoholism rested more on untested assumptions and clinical impressions than it did on fact.

It is not clear that the exclusion of women from research studies was intentional: The absence of females from most studies conducted prior to the 1970s may simply reflect the difficulty in locating large enough samples of alcoholic women for study. The prevalence of alcoholism continues to be

W. M. Cox (Ed.). *Identifying and Measuring Alcoholic Personality Characteristics.* New Directions for Methodology of Social and Behavioral Science, no. 16. San Francisco: Jossey-Bass, June 1983.

higher among men than it is among women, by ratios that vary from about eleven to one in prison samples to nearly one to one in private practitioners' offices (Schuckit and Morrissey, 1976; U.S. Department of Health and Human Services, 1981). In addition, it is often claimed that alcoholic women are more likely than alcoholic men to drink alone at home and to be sheltered by their families from the consequences of problem drinking. If this is so, it seems reasonable that fewer women would be available for study. Finally, the stigma attached to drunkenness is greater for women than it is for men, and this may have contributed to women's reluctance to seek treatment and to be available as research subjects (Sandmaier, 1980).

There is some evidence, however, that the bias of early research against female alcoholics was not only practical but in part prejudicial. Alcoholism in women has frequently been examined not as a phenomenon worthy of study for its own sake, "but as a comparison of women to the most frequently utilized yardstick of alcoholism—the male alcoholic" (Schuckit and Morrissey, 1976, p. 9). As recently as 1976, a review article on the offspring of alcoholics (El-Guebaly and Offord, 1976) contended that daughters of alcoholics were "also" important to study. The authors noted that daughters are greatly underrepresented in research studies "despite the fact that as future wives and mothers their impact is as important as that of their male counterparts" (El-Guebaly and Offord, 1976, p. 363). One major reason for concern about alcoholism in women, these authors seem to imply, is that it can impair their functioning as wives and mothers. Whether they become wives and mothers or not, women are clearly at risk for the development of a wide range of alcohol-related problems, and as such it is important to study them in their own right.

Only in the past decade has the issue of gender differences in alcoholism been addressed in a meaningful way. This new interest has resulted from growing public concern about alcoholism among women and from a concomitant increase in research on women. Despite the increased number of studies, however, many studies of alcoholic women and of gender differences in alcoholism have serious methodological flaws. Many studies—of both women and men—have employed small, nonrepresentative samples, and they have failed to provide adequate nonalcoholic control groups. Most studies have relied on case history material from clinical samples of alcoholics. Very few studies have attempted to obtain in-depth information from nonclinical samples of problem drinkers in the general population. Even fewer have employed longitudinal, experimental, or quasi-experimental designs that might permit us to draw inferences about cause and effect.

This chapter reexamines traditional notions about the female alcoholic in light of the methodological limitations of earlier research and summarizes available data on differences between male and female alcoholics in personality attributes and life experiences. Since most studies of alcoholic personality characteristics have dealt primarily or exclusively with males, an analysis of gender differences requires special attention to recent studies of females. For this reason, and because other chapters in this volume review research on male alcoholics, this chapter places the emphasis on research findings about women.

Gender Differences in Patterns and Symptoms of Alcoholism

Many of the available data on gender differences come from clinical studies that compare samples of male and female alcoholics in treatment. This research has reported male–female differences in drinking practices and consequences, in the onset and course of alcoholism, in concomitant psychosocial difficulties, and in premorbid psychopathology.

Drinking Practices and Consequences. Alcoholic men on the average report earlier and more frequent alcohol use and higher alcohol consumption on each drinking occasion than alcoholic women do. Relative to men, alcoholic women favor hard liquor and wine over beer, they are less likely to drink in the morning, and they are more likely to abuse prescription drugs in addition to alcohol (Gomberg, 1979; Mulford, 1977; Schuckit and Morrissey, 1976). However, since male alcoholics in research studies have often come from lower-class (such as state hospital) samples and female alcoholics have often been middle-class, some of the apparent gender differences may reflect the uncontrolled influence of socioeconomic status (Schuckit and Morrissey, 1976).

Socioeconomic differences and differences in traditional sex roles may also help to explain the common finding that alcoholic women tend both to conceal their drinking (which is more likely to occur in their own homes) and to be protected from its consequences (Beckman, 1975; Wanberg and Horn, 1970). Even when socioeconomic status is controlled, men are more likely than women to run afoul of the law while intoxicated, and men may be more likely than women to be arrested and prosecuted (Lisansky, 1957; Rimmer and others, 1971; Wanberg and Horn, 1970). Male alcoholics also report a higher rate of automobile accidents while drinking (Rimmer and others, 1971) and more drinking-related job impairment (Horn and Wanberg, 1973).

Onset and Course of Alcoholism. Both Lisansky (1957) and recent investigators have reported that although women begin drinking later in life than men do, they begin to experience alcohol-related difficulties in a briefer time period and hence enter treatment at approximately the same age as men. This telescoping of symptoms has been interpreted to mean that alcohol problems progress more rapidly for women than they do for men (Beckman, 1975; Gomberg, 1976). However, the similarity of age between men and women at treatment entry does not necessarily imply alcohol problems of equal severity. Rather, it may be that women are more likely than men to seek treatment at an earlier stage of alcoholism, perhaps because women's social support systems deteriorate more rapidly than those of men during the process of becoming alcoholic or because women generally are more inclined to seek professional help than men are (Beckman and Amaro, 1983). Further, it may be that the telescoping of symptoms is characteristic only of alcoholic women from upper socioeconomic strata, not descriptive of alcoholic women in general (Schuckit and Morrissey, 1976).

Concomitant Psychosocial Difficulties. The early clinical literature appeared to support the notion that alcoholic women had greater psychosocial difficulties than alcoholic men. For example, numerous studies claimed or demonstrated higher rates of broken marriages, psychiatric treatment, suicide attempts, and marriage to other alcoholics among alcoholic women than among alcoholic men (Beckman, 1975; Gomberg, 1974, 1976). However, these findings need to be interpreted with caution. Several of the behaviors in question, including marital problems and psychiatric treatment, may reflect different social reactions to the drinking problems of men and women, not preexisting gender differences in psychological disturbance. Furthermore, with regard to suicide, while the rates of attempted suicide are higher for female than for male alcoholics, the different rates may simply parallel gender differences in the general population, where the female-to-male ratio of suicide attempts is approximately three to one, not gender differences specific to alcoholism. However, a recent review by Hill (1983) suggests that alcoholic women may also be at higher risk than alcoholic men for completed suicide, which is less common among women than among men in the general population.

In any case, even if higher rates of psychological disturbance among alcoholic women than among men were confirmed by rigorous studies, the findings would need to be interpreted cautiously: "Does alcoholism cause more psychiatric disorder in women? *Or* does a woman have to be more 'ill' to overcome the more intense social stigma against heavy drinking and demonstrate alcoholism? *Or* do women displaying alcoholism more frequently have other major psychiatric disorders of which alcohol problems are symptomatic? *Or* is psychiatric disorder in women alcoholics the result of the severe social sanctions taken against women who abuse alcohol?" (Schuckit and Morrissey, 1976, p. 11).

Premorbid Psychopathology. The relationship between alcoholism and preexisting psychiatric disorders has received increasing attention in the research literature during the past decade (Schuckit and others, 1969; Winokur and others, 1970). Subgroups of alcoholics have been based on prior psychiatric diagnosis, and there are different proportions of males and females in the various subgroups. Alcoholic women in one sizable subgroups (25–30 percent) had affective disorders before they became alcoholic, while a similar percentage of alcoholic men had sociopathic disorders before they became alcoholic. A number of writers have noted that the different rates at which males and females develop these particular psychiatric disorders are true not only for future alcoholics but for the general population as well. Nevertheless, identifying the alcoholic's premorbid psychopathology may have important implications for treatment and prognosis (Braiker, 1983; Schuckit and Winokur, 1972).

Gender Differences in Life Experience Risk Factors for Alcoholism

Wall's (1937, p. 952) assertion that alcohol abuse is "more intimately associated with a definite life situation" in women than in men received support from an early clinical study by Lisansky (1957) and from several subsequent investigations (Cramer and Blacker, 1963; Curlee, 1969, 1970; Morrissey and Schuckit, 1978; Mulford, 1977). Life experiences that appear to increase the risk of alcoholism can be grouped into two major categories: experiences that occur early in life as part of the alcoholic's family of origin and experiences that occur close in time to the onset of the drinking problem and that appear to act as immediate precipitants. A third category, sexual experience and reproductive disorders, includes both childhood and adult experiences. We discuss the third category separately because of its prominence in the recent literature on alcoholism.

Early Life Events. Both alcoholic men and alcoholic women report high rates of disruption early in life. Parental absence or unavailability is frequently the source of this disruption, which includes loss of one or both parents through death, divorce, or separation and psychiatric problems, such as psychosis or alcoholism, in parents or other close relatives. Although both female and male alcoholics report higher rates of early family disruption than women and men in the general population do, alcoholic women appear to report even more such experiences than alcoholic men (Gomberg, 1980).

A possible explanation for this gender difference is that women are more sensitive than men to changes in interpersonal relationships and that they are therefore more likely to recall early disruptions in family relationships. However, it may also be that women who lose a parent or live with an alcoholic or psychotic parent are more strongly affected by the experience than men are and that they are more likely to develop alcoholism or other psychiatric disorders later in life as a result. Termination or disruption of significant early relationships may help to explain the depression and low self-esteem often noted in alcoholic women (Beckman, 1978a; Schuckit and Morrissey, 1976). The enduring feelings of loss, sadness, and anger in such women are important issues for psychotherapy to address (Wilsnack, 1982a).

Recent Stressors as Precipitants. Although the data are not completely consistent, a number of studies have found that female alcoholics are more likely than male alcoholics to link the onset of their drinking problem to a particular crisis or stressful event (Beckman, 1975; Gomberg, 1976). Events cited frequently by women include abortions, the birth of a child, divorce, health problems, children leaving home, menopause, and death in the family.

It is plausible that stressful life events contribute to alcoholism more among women than they do among men. However, it also is possible that, since the social stigma of alcohol abuse is greater for women than it is for men, women feel a greater need to rationalize or explain their deviation from expected behavior in terms of some real, external "cause." Still another possibility, mentioned in the preceding section, is that women are more sensitive to interpersonal relationships in general than men are and that they may therefore be more likely to remember and report the specific interpersonal stressors that preceded their problem drinking than men are. Several studies currently in progress are addressing these various explanations. If life stress does play a causal role in women's drinking, then some groups of women, such as those recently widowed or divorced, should be at especially high risk for alcohol abuse. Preventive efforts might be especially worthwhile with these high-risk groups.

Studies supporting the hypothesis that recent stressful life events are more causally important in the onset of drinking problems among women than they are among men have five methodological problems in common. First, Lisansky (1957) and others have urged caution in interpreting data on life stress and drinking, since women may simply be more apt to recall affect-laden events and to engage in post hoc rationalizations than men are. Not only have previous studies of life stress and drinking used self-reports, but most have merely recorded subjects' unstructured free recall of their life stresses and drinking history rather than prompting their subjects' memories with enumerated specific stresses that might be related to the onset of their drinking problem.

Second, the time period over which a stressor might be expected to exert its impact has not been controlled in these studies. For example, a woman whose alcoholism developed five years postpartum was not differentiated from a woman whose alcoholic symptoms began five weeks postpartum. In both cases, the researchers held childbirth responsible for the woman's alcoholism if the woman associated childbirth with her symptomatic drinking.

Third, the literature tends not to take the qualitative differences among various stresses into account. For example, continuous stressors, such as marital difficulties, have not been distinguished from discrete, traumatic life events, such as the death of a spouse.

Fourth, all people are not equally at risk for potentially stressful life events or for the development of alcoholism in response to such events. For example, older people are more likely than younger people to have experienced the death of a parent. Thus, if we assume that the entire population is at risk for the development of alcohol problems as a result of the death of a parent, the impact of this particular stressor as a precipitant for alcohol abuse is considerably diminished. Specifying the segment of the population that is potentially vulnerable to the impact of a particular stressor is always necessary with high-risk methodology (Heller and others, 1982).

Fifth, implicit in the life stress and alcoholism literature is the idea that many of the stresses reported are by their very nature either events that only women can experience or events that can be expected to have greater impact on women than on men. Examples of these stresses include abortion, childbirth, hysterectomy, and the "empty nest." However, it seems certain that men, too, react to such events as an abortion or a child's leaving home. Restricting the significance of these events to women has precluded systematic efforts to compare male and female alcoholics' reactions to such experiences.

A recent well-designed study (Morrissey, 1980) points up many defects of the early research. This study failed to support the earlier notion that life stress has more impact on the drinking of women than it does on the drinking of men. Morrissey sought to determine whether women are more likely than men to begin experiencing alcohol-related problems as a consequence of the birth of a child. Her careful methodology, in which a single, discrete life event was examined for its relationship to the onset of alcohol problems in both men and women, is difficult to compare directly with previous work. Nonetheless, because Morrissey's study avoided many of the pitfalls just discussed, we describe it here in some detail.

Morrissey administered the same structured interview to male and female alcoholics in a detoxification center. She not only limited the type of event inquired about but also limited the period of time during which the stressor was expected to exert its impact to two years. She was concerned only with whether a child was born, not with the parent's subjective impression of the stressfulness of the birth. Her findings indicate that there was a statistically significant gender difference in the impact of this stressor on the development of alcoholism, with births being more strongly related to alcoholism among men than they were among women. The results show that, among those who were at risk for first abusing alcohol during the two-year period following the birth of a child, men were more likely than women to become alcoholic during this period.

It is important to note that Morrissey would not have noted this gender difference if she had not added the "still at risk" qualification. Since men on the average become alcoholic earlier in life than women do, more of the men in Morrissey's sample were already alcoholic at the time of the child's birth. However, of the men who were still at risk for alcoholism more became alcoholic within the two years following the birth than the women still at risk.

Morrissey's study shows how the methodological limitations of past research may have led researchers to conclude that stressful events are more closely related to the development of alcoholism in women than they are in men. Nevertheless, we must interpret Morrissey's results cautiously for two reasons: First, only one life event was studied. Second, at least one alternative hypothesis has not been ruled out: the possibility that the birth of a child coincides with a period of generally higher risk for alcoholism among men. Since women on the average develop alcoholism after their peak childbearing years but men become alcoholic relatively early in life (Dahlgren, 1979; Winokur and Clayton, 1968), the correlation between childbirth and onset of alcoholism may be in part an artifact of gender differences in the natural history of alcoholism. Thus, until Morrissey's improved methodology has been used to study other life events and until gender differences in the natural history of alcoholism have been taken into account, we cannot conclude that stressful life events have less impact on the development of alcohol problems among women than they do among men.

Sexual Orientation, Sexual Dysfunction, and Reproductive Disorders. In a very early paper on the psychological relationship between alcoholism and sexuality, Karl Abraham (1927 [1908], p. 89) wrote that "alcoholism, sexuality, and neurosis are connected in many ways." Although the difficulties of both alcoholic men and alcoholic women have been related to their sexuality, the major focus with men has been on their sexual orientation, with a less frequent emphasis on sexual dysfunctions due to alcohol. In contrast, the primary emphasis with women who are alcoholic has been on problems of "sexual adjustment," which has been defined to include inadequate sexual and reproductive functioning on a physical level, dissatisfaction with traditional feminine sex roles, and, most recently, lesbianism and a history of sexual abuse.

Homosexuality and alcoholism have long been linked in the psychiatric literature, especially among males (Abraham, 1927 [1908]; Knight, 1937; Machover and others, 1959). Explanations for the presumed association have ranged from psychoanalytic conceptualizations of homosexuality and alcoholism as coincident oral neuroses (Bergler, 1944) to psychosocial formulations in which alcoholism is a response to society's stigmatization of the homosexual (Fifield, 1975).

The earliest studies of the coincidence of alcoholism and homosexuality, which amounted to clinical impressions published as case histories, were greatly influenced by psychoanalytic theory. More recently, survey methods have been used to estimate the rates of alcoholism in specific homosexual populations. For example, Fifield (1975) estimated that 30 percent of the male and female homosexual population in one West Coast city were either alcohol abusers or alcohol-dependent. Surveys of homosexual men in four Midwestern communities (Lohrenz and others, 1978) yielded the same estimate (30 percent) and offered further support for the belief that alcoholism and homosexuality are somehow linked. Several recent studies of women report elevated rates of homosexuality and bisexuality among female alcoholics and higher rates of alcohol problems among lesbians than among heterosexual women in the general population (Wilsnack, 1983).

Homosexual persons may experience an increased risk of developing alcoholism for a number of reasons: heavy drinking norms within many homosexual groups, the role of the gay bar as a social meeting ground, and, perhaps most significantly, the alientation, isolation, and low self-esteem that many homosexuals experience as a result of their stigmatization by society. However, methodological problems abound in this area—in particular, difficulties in obtaining representative homosexual samples and in selecting appropriate heterosexual control groups—and the nature of the relationship between alcohol abuse and sexual orientation is far from clear (Hastings, 1982; Nardi, 1982).

Besides addressing questions of sexual orientation, the recent literature on alcoholic women has explored relationships between sexual dysfunction and gynecological disorders and women's drinking. Two reviews of epidemiological and clinical studies (Wilsnack, 1982b, 1983) found consistently high rates of both sexual problems and reproductive problems among alcoholic and problem-drinking women. Rates of sexual inhibition, impaired sexual responsiveness, and anorgasmia in eighteen samples of alcoholic women ranged between 23 and 100 percent. Most of these studies reviewed lacked nonalcoholic control groups. In the few studies that included adequate controls, the rates of sexual dysfunction were higher among alcoholic women than they were among nonalcoholic women. Sixteen studies found that rates of gynecological and obstetrical problems, including dysmenorrhea, hysterectomy, early menopause, infertility, spontaneous abortion, complications in labor and delivery, and stillbirths were higher among alcoholic women than they were among women in the general population.

A primary drawback of this research is that cause and effect are difficult to unravel, since the women who became alcoholic have not been studied longitudinally. Thus, sexual and reproductive difficulties may either predate and somehow contribute to alcoholism, or they may be a consequence of it. One clear consequence of alcohol abuse for reproductive functioning is the fetal alcohol syndrome and other fetal alcohol effects (Abel, 1982; Little and Ervin, 1983). Moreover, the few studies that have tried to assess the sequence of sexual, reproductive, and alcohol problems retrospectively have found that alcoholic women report high rates of sexual, obstetrical, and gynecological problems both before and after their problem drinking begins. If these findings can be replicated with stronger (such as longitudinal) designs, they may suggest a reciprocal relationship between sexual or reproductive dysfunction and excessive drinking, in which sexual or reproductive problems both contribute to and result from heavy drinking. The findings would also be consistent with a causal pattern in which some third condition, such as a biological predisposition, traumatic early sexual experiences, or chronic psychological or environmental stress, contributes to both alcohol abuse and sexual or reproductive disorders.

The role of sexual abuse has received increasing attention as a possible precursor of alcohol and sexual problems among women. Clinical and anecdotal evidence (reviewed by Wilsnack, 1983) strongly supports the impression that many women who become alcoholic have been sexually abused in a variety of ways, including incest, rape, and other traumata. Nevertheless, better time-ordered data from both alcoholic and general population samples are needed if we are to determine more precisely the impact that these sexual traumata may have on future sexual dysfunction and alcohol problems among women.

Motivations for Drinking: Power and Dependence

Men's motivations for drinking received considerable research attention in the 1960s and early 1970s, which led to several theories about the motivational bases of alcohol use and abuse. Using various research methods, including laboratory analogues, administration of Thematic Apperception Tests (TATs) at experimental drinking parties, and cross-cultural analyses of folktales and ethnographic ratings, McClelland and his colleagues (McClelland and others, 1972) reached the conclusion that a man's concern with power plays a pivotal role in determining how much he is likely to drink. The power theory of drinking that emerged from these studies posits that drinking gratifies needs for feelings of personal power over others. Two kinds of power were distinguished: socialized power, which was defined as the use of power on behalf of other people, as in teaching or helping others, and personalized power, which was described as a more selfish power orientation, as reflected, for example, in TAT themes that emphasize competition and victory, sexual exploitation, domination, and physical aggression. Among male drinkers, feelings of socialized power increased with low to moderate levels of drinking, while feelings of personalized power increased at higher levels of consumption.

Because men traditionally have been socialized to be concerned about their personal power and because they are more likely than women to experience social demands to display power and control, they may be more likely than women to desire the temporary feelings of power produced by alcohol. Indeed, two studies of female social drinkers (described by Wilsnack, 1976) found that drinking decreased several traditionally masculine characteristics and that it increased several traditionally feminine characteristics of women's thoughts. As discussed more fully later in this chapter, these findings suggest that drinking by both men and women leads to psychological states that are consistent with traditional sex-role stereotypes (Frieze and Schafer, 1983; Scoufis and Walker, 1982).

Power needs as a motive for drinking were discrepant with the previous literature, which had concluded that desires for dependence and nurturance were the primary motives for drinking among men (Bacon and others, 1965; Lisansky, 1960; McCord and McCord, 1960). The dependence theory of alcoholism, as articulated by Blane (1968) and others, maintains that drinking gratifies dependence needs by enabling the drinker to feel warm, sentimental, and close to others. At the same time, the drinker can maintain a facade of maturity and self-sufficiency due to the social definition of drinking as an adult, masculine behavior. Blane believed that male alcoholics could be classified by the way in which their dependence needs are manifested: The counterdependent alcoholic denies his unconscious dependence needs and acts very independently while sober; the passive-dependent alcoholic expresses his needs for warmth, help, and nurturance openly, whether he is drinking or not; while the dependent/independent alcoholic vacillates between extreme independence and dependence. According to Blane's formulation, men are more prone to drink than women are because of society's greater intolerance of men's overt expression of dependence needs. Women who abuse alcohol in spite of society's greater permissiveness of their emotional expressiveness and dependent behavior presumably either have decreased opportunity for gratifying their dependence needs, or they have unusually intense dependence needs in the first place. Some observers (Barry, 1976) have noted that the power and dependence theories may simply be two complementary views of the same process, in which overt power needs arise in reaction to underlying feelings of weakness and dependence.

Self-Concept and Self-Esteem

The findings of a number of studies indicate that negative self-image and low self-esteem are associated with alcohol abuse for both men and women. Studies consistently report that alcoholic men show less favorable self-concept and lower self-esteem than nonalcoholic men and men with other psychiatric disorders (Cox, 1979). Alcoholic women have been found to view themselves as less personally competent, to have significantly poorer self-concept, and to report greater anxiety than nonalcoholic women do (McLachlan and others, 1979). There is also evidence that problem drinking among college males is associated with negative self-concept, anxiety, and depression (Williams, 1966) and that college-age women who drink heavily perceive that they are motivated to do so more by feelings of powerlessness and inadequacy than by wishes to be sociable (Beckman and Bardsley, 1981).

A few studies have directly compared the self-esteem of male and female alcoholics. Clarke (1974) found no difference in self-esteem between twenty alcoholic men and twenty alcoholic women. However, a larger, well-controlled study by Beckman (1978a) found that alcoholic women scored lower on self-esteem than both nonalcoholic women and alcoholic men. Finally, Heilbrun and Schwartz (1980) found that, although alcoholic men were lower in self-esteem than alcoholic women, the alcoholic men were also more effective rationalizers of their own behavior. Heilbrun and Schwartz (1980, p. 1134) hypothesized that at least some alcoholic men may "neutralize their deficit in self-esteem" via an enhanced self-reinforcement ability manifested in their greater capacity to rationalize their own unacceptable behaviors.

Although it has been clearly demonstrated that a prominent personality characteristic of alcoholics is their low self-esteem, it is unclear whether this poor self-image precedes alcoholism or whether it is a consequence of alcoholism. It is generally believed that alcoholics drink in order to bolster their feelings of confidence and adequacy, but evidence from several studies fails to support this view (Pollack, 1965; Vanderpool, 1969). A recent study by Konovsky and Wilsnack (1982) found that self-satisfaction actually decreased in nonalcoholic women after moderate drinking in a natural party setting. People who drink tend to expect positive effects from alcohol, regardless of its actual effects (Brown and others, 1980). Thus, persons with low self-esteem may believe that drinking will help them to feel better about themselves. If they do not get the expected relief from self-disapproval from drinking, a vicious circle may begin in which low self-esteem leads to increased drinking, which lowers self-esteem even more.

Sex Roles and Sex-Role Conflicts

Sex Roles and Alcohol Abuse Among Women. Recent studies suggest that conflicts surrounding traditional feminine roles may be more common among problem-drinking and alcoholic women than they are among women in general. These conflicts have taken two major forms. In one form, there is an inconsistency between the woman's sex-role attitudes and values and her actual behavior. Such a woman might espouse traditionally feminine attitudes and values while engaging in nontraditional role behavior (Beckman, 1978b; Wilsnack, 1976). In the other form, which has been described in the research literature less frequently but which has often been reported by clinicians, the discrepancy is not between the woman's own sex-role attitudes and behavior but between her sex-role orientation and the demands of her social environment. For example, the significant others of an assertive, independent woman may expect her to behave in sex-stereotyped, passive-dependent ways (Sandmaier, 1980). Results from a 1975 survey (Johnson, 1982) may illustrate either or both of these forms of sex-role conflict or simply the stress created by combining multiple roles: This survey found that married women employed outside the home had higher rates of heavy and problem drinking than either unmarried employed women or married women not employed outside the home. Other data (Richardson, 1981) suggest that rigid endorsement of sex-stereotyped personality traits by either sex (that is, of traditional masculine traits by men or of traditional feminine traits by women) is associated with increased risk for problem drinking and alcoholism. In contrast, psychological androgyny (flexible integration of traditional masculine and traditional feminine traits) is associated with reduced risk.

Problem drinking can result from sex-role conflicts in at least two ways: The woman with a sex-role conflict may reduce or attempt to reduce the accompanying stress and tension by drinking alcohol, and drinking itself may serve to express sex-role values—for example, the endorsement of traditional masculine roles or the rejection of traditional feminine roles. In addition, traditional sex roles can affect drinking opportunities and exposure to drinking situations (Leland, 1981; Wilsnack and Wilsnack, 1979). Further research is needed to determine the prevalence of sex-role-related reasons for drinking among alcoholic and problem-drinking women. One study by Beckman (1978b) suggests that as many as 25 percent of alcoholic women experience internal psychological sex-role conflicts. In addition, more information is needed about how both intrapsychic and person-environment sex-role conflicts interact with other biological and psychosocial factors that increase women's risk for alcohol abuse.

Moreover, the recent studies suggesting that sex-role conflicts are related to women's drinking problems need to be interpreted cautiously. The explanatory concepts offered in these studies, such as "unconscious masculinity" and "conscious hyperfemininity," need to be described and operationalized in ways that do not reinforce negative sex-role stereotypes. Furthermore, age, socioeconomic, and ethnic differences in sex-role attitudes and behaviors may be so great that separate sex-role measures should be developed for various demographic subgroups (Leland, 1981). Finally, it is important to determine whether and in what ways the sex-role conflicts of alcoholic women differ from those of women with other psychiatric disorders.

Sex Roles, Power, and Alcohol Abuse Among Men. Surely, if sex-role factors figure in the development of alcoholism among some women, we should consider the possibility that they also relate to alcohol abuse among men. Are men who drink as a form of traditional masculine role-playing—that is, to act and feel like a man—at increased risk for heavy alcohol use and alcohol problems (Wilsnack and Wilsnack, 1979, 1980)? Can alcohol abuse be a risk among men who assume nontraditional roles? For example, are today's newly emerging househusbands conflicted over their stereotypically gender-inappropriate roles? If they are, can we expect to see an increase in alcohol abuse among this subgroup of male drinkers who are shouldering new domestic responsibilities, particularly among those who are internally or interpersonally conflicted about their new role?

If we reexamine McClelland's (McClelland and others, 1972) distinction between socialized and personalized power in light of the new rhetoric of sex roles and androgyny, it appears that the altruistic, social power needs can be reframed as an expression of a maternal, nurturant, traditionally feminine orientation. Similarly, the personal power needs that seem to be gratified when men drink heavily epitomize the sterotypical, self-assertive, masculine male. Consequently, one function of alcohol use for males who are conflicted about needs or tendencies that deviate from cultural stereotypes of masculinity may be to reduce this discrepancy. For example, both men who are consciously masculine but unconsciously less masculine and men who are conflicted about "unmasculine" dependence needs may find that drinking helps them to feel more congruent with cultural and societal expectations. Abraham (1927 [1908], p. 86) made essentially the same observation seventy-five years ago: "Men turn to alcohol because it gives them an increased feeling of manliness and flatters their complex of masculinity." Abraham's conclusion about men parallels more recent observations discussed in this chapter that the reverse process seems to hold for some women with drinking problems. These women might be said to drink in order to flatter their complex of femininity.

Viewed in this way, power as a motive for men's drinking is analogous to the sex-role factors that relate to the development of drinking problems in at least some women. For some male and female alcoholics, one function that alcohol use seems to serve is to enhance the sense that they are conforming to the sex-role expectations dictated by society.

Social Roles in Transition. Sex-role influences, whether for alcoholic men or women, can and should be viewed in a larger context, not merely as intrapsychic conflicts but also as a societal issue reflecting a social order in transition. For example, while changes in women's occupational and family roles since World War II have given many women new options and opportunities, they have also created questions, conflicts, and new demands. The choice for many women today is between two extremes: trying to lead an androgynous, superwoman life (combining occupational, marital, and family roles that typically involve overwork, overextension, and exhaustion) or, equally difficult, trying to fulfill a 1950s traditional wife–mother role in a 1980s world that expects "more" of women. What is the influence of this social upheaval on alcoholism and other forms of psychopathology in women? A sociohistorical analysis of recent changes in the roles of women and men is a critical matrix within which we can begin to think about problem behaviors and symptoms that in the past have been thought of as personality variables. Such behaviors may be unrecognized artifacts of cultural expectations and cultural change.

The composite picture that emerges from the recent literature on female alcoholics is that of a woman who is uncertain or conflicted about her womanliness, who has little self-esteem, who has no clear sense of identity, and who may be experiencing depression as well as alcoholism. This picture appears to be especially accurate for women whose alcohol problems surface later in life. From a sociohistorical perspective, these characteristics may say less about what it means to be an alcoholic woman than they do about the stresses inherent in being a woman at this time in history. Further research is needed on longitudinal changes in the drinking behavior of both men and women during this period of sex-role change. Such research can help to clarify the effects on drinking of recent changes in the roles of men and women and explicate relationships among sex-role influences and other antecedents of drinking and drinking problems.

Conclusions

Despite the many similarities between alcoholic men and women, gender differences have been reported in a variety of alcoholic personality characteristics and life experiences. This chapter has reviewed cross-gender similarities and differences in the onset and course of alcoholism, concomitant and premorbid psychopathology, life experience risk factors, motivations for drinking, self-concept and self-esteem, and social role influences.

The studies reviewed here have a variety of methodological limitations, including small and nonrepresentative samples, lack of attention to subgroup differences, absence of control groups, and lack of longitudinal data. In order to remedy these inadequacies and expand our knowledge of gender differences in alcoholism, four areas seem to have high priority for future research.

Attention to Subgroup Differences. One major contribution of the studies reviewed here has been to demonstrate that alcoholic women as a group differ from alcholic men as a group in a number of personality characteristics and life experiences. For this reason, one important task of future research will be to examine gender differences and similarities within various demographic and clinical subgroupings. Potentially important subgroups include those based on sociodemographic characteristics, such as age, ethnicity, and socioeconomic status; prior psychiatric diagnosis; and antecedents of drinking, such as persons with and without a family history of alcoholism and persons with and without precipitating stressful life events. Subgroup analyses will help to clarify the possible confounding influences of various background characteristics, such as socioeconomic status, in previous research, and it will allow treatment and prevention programs to be targeted more precisely to both gender-related characteristics and to other subgroup-related characteristics of clients.

Specificity of Drinking Behavior. Most studies discussed in this chapter have compared alcoholic men and women with nonalcoholic persons from the general population, if indeed they have included control groups at all. Thus, it is not clear whether the personality characteristics identified are specific to alcoholism or whether they also apply to men and women who have other types of psychiatric disorders and addictive behaviors. Since many alcoholics also abuse psychoactive drugs, it seems possible that their personality manifestations are characteristic of addiction-prone individuals in general. Hence, future research should explore the role that specific personality factors, such as attitudes toward alcohol and other psychoactive drugs, and social factors, such as peer influences and drinking or drug use opportunities, play in the particular type of addictive behavior that is acquired. To answer these various questions, future studies will have to include control groups of men and women with psychiatric disorders and addictive behaviors other than alcoholism in addition to control groups consisting of normal individuals.

Interdisciplinary Research Involving Complex Models. This chapter has focused on gender differences in individual personality variables, including psychiatric symptomatology, drinking motivations, self-concept and self-esteem, and sex-role adoption. However, a wide variety of biological and sociocultural variables may also contribute to the development of alcoholism, in ways that may be similar or different for men and women. One important task for the future is to develop complex multivariate models to guide interdisciplinary research on the interaction of personality characteristics with biological predispositions and with various sociocultural antecedents of alcohol abuse and alcoholism.

Importance of Longitudinal Data. As noted throughout this chapter, the lack of longitudinal data—or even of retrospective time-ordered data—is a serious limitation of the existing research on gender differences in alcoholism. As in other areas of alcoholism research, longitudinal studies of nonalcoholic and prealcoholic men and women are needed if we are to address the important questions about cause and effect that the cross-sectional clinical studies that make up most of the available literature leave unanswered.

Further research on gender differences in alcoholism seems clearly warranted. Finding similarities in personality characteristics and other antecedents and consequences of alcoholism between alcoholic men and women will allow the accumulated findings of earlier research on men to be applied to women as well. Finding gender differences will allow alcoholism treatment and prevention programs to be tailored to the special characteristics and needs of both men and women.

References

Abel, E. L. (Ed.). *Fetal Alcohol Syndrome.* Boca Raton, Fla.: CRC Press, 1982.

Abraham, K. "The Psychological Relations Between Sexuality and Alcoholism." In *Selected Papers of Karl Abraham, M.D.* New York: Brunner/Mazel, 1927. (Originally published 1908.)

Bacon, M. K., Barry, H., and Child, I. L. "A Cross-Cultural Study of Drinking. II. Relations to Other Features of Culture." *Quarterly Journal of Studies on Alcohol,* 1965, Supplement No. 3, 29–48.

Barry, H. "Cross-Cultural Evidence That Dependency Conflict Motivates Drunkenness." In M. W. Everett, J. O. Waddell, and D. B. Heath (Eds.), *Cross-Cultural Approaches to the Study of Alcohol: An Interdisciplinary Perspective.* The Hague: Mouton, 1976.

Beckman, L. J. Women Alcoholics: A Review of Social and Psychological Studies." *Journal of Studies on Alcohol,* 1975, *36* (7), 797–824.

Beckman, L. J. "Self-Esteem of Women Alcoholics." *Journal of Studies on Alcohol,* 1978a, *39* (3), 491–498.

Beckman, L. J. "Sex-Role Conflict in Alcoholic Women: Myth or Reality." *Journal of Abnormal Psychology,* 1978b, *87* (4), 408–417.

Beckman, L. J., and Amaro, H. "Patterns of Women's Use of Alcohol Treatment Agencies." In S. C. Wilsnack and L. J. Beckman (Eds.), *Alcohol Problems in Women: Antecedents, Consequences, and Intervention.* New York: Guilford, 1983.

Beckman, L. J., and Bardsley, P. E. "The Perceived Determinants and Consequences of Alcohol Consumption Among Young Women Heavy Drinkers." *International Journal of the Addictions,* 1981, *16* (1), 75–88.

Bergler, E. "Contributions to the Psychogenesis of Alcohol Addiction." *Quarterly Journal of Studies on Alcohol,* 1944, *5,* 434–449.

Blane, H. T. *The Personality of the Alcoholic: Guises of Dependency.* New York: Harper & Row, 1968.

Braiker, H. B. "Therapeutic Issues in the Treatment of Alcoholic Women." In S. C. Wilsnack and L. J. Beckman (Eds.), *Alcohol Problems in Women: Antecedents, Consequences, and Intervention.* New York: Guilford, 1983.

Brown, S. A., and others. "Expectations of Reinforcement from Alcohol: Their Domain and Relation to Drinking Patterns." *Journal of Consulting and Clinical Psychology,* 1980, *48* (4), 419–426.

Clarke, S. K. "Self-Esteem in Men and Women Alcoholics." *Quarterly Journal of Studies on Alcohol,* 1974, *35* (4), 1380–1381.

Cox, W. M. "The Alcoholic Personality: A Review of the Evidence." In B. A. Maher (Ed.), *Progress in Experimental Personality Research.* Vol. 9. New York: Academic Press, 1979.

Cramer, M. J., and Blacker, E. "'Early' and 'Late' Problem Drinkers Among Female Prisoners." *Journal of Health and Human Behavior,* 1963, *4,* 282–290.

Curlee, J. "Alcoholism and the 'Empty Nest.'" *Bulletin of the Menninger Clinic,* 1969, *33* (3), 165–171.

Curlee, J. "A Comparison of Male and Female Patients at an Alcoholic Treatment Center." *Journal of Psychology,* 1970, *74,* 239–247.

Dahlgren, L. *Female Alcoholics: A Psychiatric and Social Study.* Stockholm: Karolinska Institute, 1979.

El-Guebaly, N., and Offord, D. R. "The Offspring of Alcoholics: A Critical Review." *American Journal of Psychiatry,* 1976, *134* (4), 357–365.

Fifield, L. *On My Way to Nowhere: Alienated, Isolated, Drunk.* Los Angeles: Gay Community Services Center, 1975.

Frieze, I. H., and Schafer, P. C. "Alcohol Use and Marital Violence: Female and Male Differences in Reactions to Alcohol." In S. C. Wilsnack and L. J. Beckman (Eds.), *Alcohol Problems in Women: Antecedents, Consequences, and Intervention.* New York: Guilford, 1983.

Gomberg, E. S. "Women and Alcoholism." In V. Franks and V. Burtle (Eds.), *Women in Therapy.* New York: Brunner/Mazel, 1974.

Gomberg, E. S. "The Female Alcoholic." In R. E. Tarter and A. A. Sugerman (Eds.), *Alcoholism: Interdisciplinary Approaches to an Enduring Problem.* Reading, Mass.: Addison-Wesley, 1976.

Gomberg, E. S. "Problems with Alcohol and Other Drugs." In E. S. Gomberg and V. Franks (Eds.), *Gender and Disordered Behavior.* New York: Brunner/Mazel, 1979.

Gomberg, E. S. "Risk Factors Related to Alcohol Problems Among Women: Proneness and Vulnerability." In *Alcoholism and Alcohol Abuse Among Women: Research Issues.* National Institute on Alcohol Abuse and Alcoholism. Research Monograph No. 1. Washington, D.C.: U.S. Government Printing Office, 1980.

Hastings, P. "Alcohol and the Lesbian Community: Changing Patterns of Awareness." *Drinking and Drug Practices Surveyor,* August 1982, pp. 3–7.

Heilbrun, A. B., Jr., and Schwartz, H. L. "Self-Esteem and Self-Reinforcement in Men Alcoholics: An Explanation of a Paradox." *Journal of Studies on Alcohol,* 1980, *41* (11), 1134–1142.

Heller, K., Sher, K., and Benson, C. "Problems Associated with Risk Overprediction in Studies of Offspring of Alcoholics: Implications for Prevention." *Clinical Psychology Review,* 1982, *2,* 183–200.

Hill, S. Y. "Vulnerability to the Biomedical Consequences of Alcholism and Alcohol-Related Problems Among Women." In S. C. Wilsnack and L. J. Beckman (Eds.), *Alcohol Problems in Women: Antecedents, Consequences, and Intervention.* New York: Guilford, 1983.

Horn, J. L., and Wanberg, K. W. "Females Are Different: On the Diagnosis of Alcoholism in Women." In *Proceedings of the First Annual Alcoholism Conference of the National Institute on Alcohol Abuse and Alcoholism.* Washington, D.C.: U.S. Government Printing Office, 1973.

Johnson, P. B. "Sex Differences, Women's Roles, and Alcohol Use: Preliminary National Data." *Journal of Social Issues,* 1982, *38* (2), 93–116.

Knight, R. P. "The Psychodynamics of Chronic Alcoholism." *Journal of Nervous and Mental Disease,* 1937, *86,* 538–548.

Konovsky, M., and Wilsnack, S. C. "Social Drinking and Self-Esteem in Married Couples." *Journal of Studies on Alcohol,* 1982, *43* (3), 319–333.

Leland, J. "Sex Roles, Family Organization, and Alcohol Abuse." In J. Orford and J. Harwin (Eds.), *Alcohol and the Family.* London: Croom Helm, 1981.

Lisansky, E. S. "Alcoholism in Women: Social and Psychological Concomitants. I. Social History Data." *Quarterly Journal of Studies on Alcohol,* 1957, *18* (4), 588–623.

Lisansky, E. S. "The Etiology of Alcoholism: The Role of Psychological Predisposition." *Quarterly Journal of Studies on Alcohol,* 1960, *21,* 314–343.

Little, R. E., and Ervin, C. H. "Alcohol Use and Reproduction." In S. C. Wilsnack and L. J. Beckman (Eds.), *Alcohol Problems in Women: Antecedents, Consequences, and Intervention.* New York: Guilford, 1983.

Lohrenz, L. J., and others. "Alcohol Problems in Several Midwestern Homosexual Communities." *Journal of Studies on Alcohol,* 1978, *39* (11), 1959–1963.

Machover, S., and others. "Clinical and Objective Studies of Personality Variables in Alcoholism. III. An Objective Study of Homosexuality and Alcoholism." *Quarterly Journal of Studies on Alcohol,* 1959, *20,* 528–542.

McClelland, D. C., and others. *The Drinking Man: Alcohol and Human Motivation.* New York: Free Press, 1972.

McCord, W., and McCord, J. *Origins of Alcoholism.* Stanford, Calif.: Stanford University Press, 1960.

McLachlan, J. F., and others. "Self-Evaluation, Role Satisfaction, and Anxiety in the Woman Alcoholic." *International Journal of the Addictions,* 1979, *14* (6), 809–832.

Morrissey, E. R. "The Role of Life Change in the Development of Alcohol-Related Problems: An Investigation of Gender Differences." Unpublished doctoral dissertation, University of Washington, 1980.

Morrissey, E. R., and Schuckit, M. A. "Stressful Life Events and Alcohol Problems Among Women Seen at a Detoxication Center." *Journal of Studies on Alcohol,* 1978, *39* (9), 1559–1576.

Mulford, H. A. "Women and Men Problem Drinkers: Sex Differences in Patients Served by Iowa's Community Alcoholism Centers." *Journal of Studies on Alcohol,* 1977, *38* (9), 1624–1639.

Nardi, P. M. "Alcoholism and Homosexuality: A Theoretical Perspective." *Journal of Homosexuality,* 1982, *7* (4), 9–25.

Pollack, D. "Experimental Intoxication of Alcoholics and Normals: Some Psychological Changes." Unpublished doctoral dissertation, University of California, 1965.

Richardson, A. M. "Androgyny: How It Affects Drinking Practices." *Focus on Women: Journal of Addictions and Health,* 1981, *2,* 116–131.

Rimmer, J., and others. "Alcoholism. II. Sex, Socioeconomic Status, and Race in Two Hospitalized Samples." *Quarterly Journal of Studies on Alcohol,* 1971, *32* (4), 942–952.

Sandmaier, M. *The Invisible Alcoholics: Women and Alcohol Abuse in America.* New York: McGraw-Hill, 1980.

Schuckit, M. A., and Morrissey, E. R. "Alcoholism in Women: Some Clinical and Social Perspectives with an Emphasis on Possible Subtypes." In M. Greenblatt and M. A. Schuckit (Eds.), *Alcoholism Problems in Women and Children.* New York: Grune & Stratton, 1976.

Schuckit, M. A., and others. "Alcoholism. I. Two Types of Alcoholism in Women." *Archives of General Psychiatry,* 1969, *20,* 301–306.

Schuckit, M. A., and Winokur, G. "A Short-Term Follow-Up of Women Alcoholics." *Diseases of the Nervous System,* 1972, *33* (10), 672–678.

Scoufis, P., and Walker, M. "Heavy Drinking and the Need for Power." *Journal of Studies on Alcohol,* 1982, *43* (9), 1010–1019.

U.S. Department of Health and Human Services, National Institute on Alcohol Abuse and Alcoholism. *Fourth Special Report to the U.S. Congress on Alcohol and Health.* Washington, D.C.: U.S. Government Printing Office, 1981.

Vanderpool, J. A. "Alcoholism and Self-Concept." *Quarterly Journal of Studies on Alcohol,* 1969, *30,* 59-77.

Wall, J. H. "A Study of Alcoholism in Women." *American Journal of Psychiatry,* 1937, *93,* 943-952.

Wanberg, K. W., and Horn, J. L. "Alcoholism Symptom Patterns of Men and Women." *Quarterly Journal of Studies on Alcohol,* 1970, *31* (1), 40-61.

Williams, A. F. "Social Drinking, Anxiety, and Depression." *Journal of Personality and Social Psychology,* 1966, *3,* 689-693.

Wilsnack, R. W., and Wilsnack, S. C. "Drinking and Denial of Social Obligations in Adolescent Boys." *Journal of Studies on Alcohol,* 1980, *41* (11), 1118-1133.

Wilsnack, S. C. "The Impact of Sex Roles on Women's Alcohol Use and Abuse." In M. Greenblatt and M. A. Schuckit (Eds.), *Alcoholism Problems in Women and Children.* New York: Grune & Stratton, 1976.

Wilsnack, S. C. "Alcohol Abuse and Alcoholism in Women." In E. M. Pattison and E. Kaufman (Eds.), *Encyclopedic Handbook of Alcoholism.* New York: Gardner Press, 1982a.

Wilsnack, S. C. "Alcohol, Sexuality, and Reproductive Dynsfunction in Women." In E. L. Abel (Ed.), *Fetal Alcohol Syndrome.* Vol. 2: *Human Studies.* Boca Raton, Fla.: CRC Press, 1982b.

Wilsnack, S. C. "Drinking, Sexuality, and Sexual Dysfunction in Women." In S. C. Wilsnack and L. J. Beckman (Eds.), *Alcohol Problems in Women: Antecedents, Consequences, and Intervention.* New York: Guilford, 1983.

Wilsnack, S. C., and Wilsnack, R. W. "Sex Roles and Adolescent Drinking." In H. T. Blane and M. E. Chafetz (Eds.), *Youth, Alcohol, and Social Policy.* New York: Plenum, 1979.

Winokur, G., and Clayton, P. "Family History Studies. IV. Comparison of Male and Female Alcoholics." *Quarterly Journal of Studies on Alcohol,* 1968, *29* (4), 885-891.

Winokur, G., and others. "Alcoholism. III. Diagnosis and Familial Psychiatric Illness in 259 Alcoholic Probands." *Archives of General Psychiatry,* 1970, *23,* 104-111.

Carole S. Benson is assistant professor of clinical psychiatry and behavioral sciences and coordinator of clinical training at Northwestern University Medical School, Division of Psychology.

Sharon C. Wilsnack is associate professor of psychology and director of preclinical curriculum in psychiatry and behavioral science at the University of North Dakota School of Medicine.

The consistently fruitless search for a unique alcoholic personality structure is finally giving way to the development of taxonomies of drinkers.

Alcoholic Personality or Personalities: Scale and Profile Data from the MMPI

Craig MacAndrew

While untutored common sense has long held that some persons drink too much, it was only in the decades after World War II that the notion that excessive recourse to alcohol may be due to disease achieved wide acceptance. Since the received wisdom now holds that some—but not all—of those who drink to obvious excess suffer from the disease of alcoholism, a criterion problem has necessarily arisen: How are true alcoholics to be distinguished from mere heavy drinkers?

The Criterion Problem

The proposal that we should apply a medical model to the phenomenon of excessive alcohol consumption has been entertained recurrently over the past two centuries. However, I have argued elsewhere (MacAndrew, 1969) that this proposal was not motivated by a concern to bring theory into better comport with newly discovered scientific findings. Indeed, it would be difficult to argue that the empirical case for a disease formulation is any better today than it was when Benjamin Rush made his now widely celebrated proposal to this effect some two centuries. Something has changed, however, for while

W. M. Cox (Ed.). *Identifying and Measuring Alcoholic Personality Characteristics.* New Directions for Methodology of Social and Behavioral Science, no. 16. San Francisco: Jossey-Bass, June 1983.

earlier efforts to gain acceptance for a disease model met with scant success, the most recent effort—an effort that for all practical purposes can be said to have started in the 1930s—has clearly carried the day. Since the hard criteria that would provide the diagnosis of alcoholism with its unequivocal empirical warrant have yet to be discovered, it can only be concluded that what has changed is the willingness of society to respond to the chronic drunkard in a new way. Functionally, as Seeley (1962) noted, the proposal that alcoholism is a disease constitutes a recommendation that, in our approach to the problems with which the chronic drunkard confronts us, we comport ourselves as if this were so, and acceptance of the proposal constitutes an agreement that we will so comport ourselves.

While acceptance of the disease formulation has produced the criterion problem to which I have alluded, the same formulation also contains the essentials for a solution to the problem. The solution runs something like this: Unless and until the quest for empirically adequate inclusion and exclusion criteria for the class *alcoholic* bears fruit, when it is said of an individual that he or she is an alcoholic or that he or she is a heavy drinker but not an alcoholic, it is a judgment that is being rendered. Specifically, it is a judgment that the individual's consumption of alcohol is (or is not) reflective of or is (or is not) caused by a disease process. Since judgments about the presence or absence of disease are the province of medicine, the solution to the criterion problem is provided by some such formulation as this: One is an alcoholic if and only if a member of the medical profession, acting in his or her capacity as a member of that profession, so determines.

Although this solution is operational in the superficial sense, it is far from ideal on several counts, not the least important of which is that members of the medical profession do not always agree in their judgments; indeed, they do not always agree with themselves from one occasion to another. Thus, the research enterprise, having increasingly committed itself to the disease model over the past few decades, has come increasingly to focus its efforts on the attempt to rectify the manifestly capricious nature of its criterion. The task with which alcoholism research (as opposed to alcohol research; that is, to research of a broadly social sort that focuses on the relationship between alcohol, individuals, and society) came to be preeminently concerned was construction of a more viable defense of the disease model. To accomplish this aim, it attempted to ascertain the specific way or ways in which persons who have been diagnosed as alcoholics differ from the rest of suffering humanity.

In this chapter, I assess the contribution that the vast body of data generated by the Minnesota Multiphasic Personality Inventory (MMPI) has made to this quest. Because relatively few MMPI data on female alcoholics have been published and because there is no particular reason to suppose that female alcoholics are similar to their male counterparts in all important respects, the discussion will be limited almost entirely to males.

The Minnesota Multiphasic Personality Inventory (MMPI)

The MMPI, constructed on the basis of a criterion group strategy, was introduced some forty years ago by S. R. Hathaway and J. C. McKinley to provide a multiphasic assessment of personality. As conventionally scored, its 550 different items—to which respondents answer true, false, or cannot say—constitute, in sundry combinations, thirteen standard scales consisting of three validity scales and ten clinical scales. Soon after the instrument was introduced, it became evident that the individual clinical scales did not possess the discriminant validity that had been expected of them. In consequence, MMPI interpretation soon abandoned its initial focus on validity and came to rely instead on codification of the myriad empirical findings that arose in piecemeal fashion from the vast body of data that accumulated on the ten clinical scales.

Critics of the MMPI have seemingly had a field day with the instrument on purely psychometric grounds. (For a defense of the MMPI, see Hathaway, 1972.) Nevertheless, the MMPI continues to be a mainstay of many psychological and psychiatric screening programs, and it remains by far the most frequently encountered source of psychological test data in the alcohol literature. How have these data contributed to explication of the presupposed uniqueness of the alcoholic personality?

The Quest for a Unique Alcoholic Personality

The search for the elements from which we can construct a unique alcoholic personality structure has produced a vast literature in which the responses of alcoholics have been compared with those of nonalcoholics on innumerable psychological instruments. But, the resulting statistically significant findings have been both so numerous and so diverse that Keller (1972, p. 1147) felt compelled to propose the following law: "The investigation of any trait in alcoholics will show that they have either more or less of it." Keller's resort to irony was occasioned not by what at first glance seems to be an embarrassment of riches but by the fact that, with very few exceptions, the assortment of statistically significant findings has failed to withstand even the most perfunctory challenge of cross-validation.

For those who use the MMPI, the first and most obvious place to look for alcoholic uniqueness is the ten clinical scales. For this reason, it is instructive to note that, in a recent, quite thorough review of the literature on alcoholic specificity from the perspective of "objective" (standardized) assessment methods, Miller (1976, p. 659) concluded that, aside from the fact that samples of alcoholics "tend to score higher on the Psychopathic deviance [sic] scale [Scale 4] of the MMPI than do most other populations, . . . there are virtually no established [psychometric] commonalities."

In an attempt to determine what accounts for the singular robustness of

Scale 4, MacAndrew and Geertsma (1963) compared the differential response rates of samples of 200 male outpatient alcoholics and 200 nonalcoholic and nondrug-abusing male psychiatric outpatients on this scale's fifty constitutive items. Later, MacAndrew (1978) compared the differential item response rates of similarly defined samples of female patients ($N = 195$ for each group). By ranking the fifty items on the basis of the magnitudes of their respective chi-squares, then by eliminating individual items until the mean *K*-corrected Scale 4 scores of the two patient groups were no longer statistically significant, it was found for both sexes that the elimination of only three items reduced the initially modest but statistically significant mean differences to nonsignificance.

Since both comparisons located the same three items (identically scored and with identical magnitude ranks), we must turn to these three items if we are to understand the robustness of Scale 4. However, we find that these items tell us nothing new. In the order in which they were eliminated, the items are: "I have used alcohol excessively" (MMPI booklet number 215; True); "I have never been in trouble with the law" (MMPI booklet number 294; False); and "I have not lived the right kind of life" (MMPI booklet number 61; True). By the reckoning of Scale 4, then, alcoholics cannot be distinguished from general runs of substance abuse–free psychiatric outpatients save in that they drink too much and they suffer unhappy consequences from so doing. So much, then, for the contribution of the MMPI clinical scales to our quest.

Since none of the MMPI clinical scales was constructed specifically to assess alcoholism, it soon occurred to some researchers that a more direct approach to the delineation of alcoholic specificity was in order. A criterion group strategy, they reasoned, would provide the most straightforward approach to the detection of any uniqueness that alcoholics might possess. The early and widely cited products of this approach are the alcoholism scales introduced by Hampton (1953), Holmes (1953; reported by Button, 1956), and Hoyt and Sedlacek (1958). Although different decision rules dictated item selection in these three scales, they were alike in that they were derived from comparisons between the item response rates of samples of diagnosed male alcoholics and the item response rates of putatively normal males. Thus, we might suppose that these scales would share an appreciable number of common items. However, examination by MacAndrew and Geertsma (1964) revealed that, while the three scales contained 191 different items, 151 items appeared on one scale only, or, if an item appeared on two or more scales, it was scored True on one scale and False on another. Only seven items appeared on all three scales with the same scoring. Since there was no obvious reason to fault the composition of the samples of putative normals that the authors used in constructing their scales—indeed, both Holmes and Hoyt and Sedlacek used the MMPI's original standardization sample of adult male normals—the absence of common items suggests that the personality structure of alcoholics might well be far less homogeneous than commonly supposed.

Subsequently, two composite alcoholism scales comprised of items common to two or more existing scales were introduced (Rich and Davis, 1969; Rosenberg, 1972). Even more recently, Atsaides and others (1977) produced an eight-item scale intended to differentiate institutionalized chronic alcoholics from hospitalized neurotics. Cross-validation data on all three scales, however, are either minimal, as in the case of the scale constructed by Atsaides and others, or they are nonexistent.

Moreover, the search for the presumed uniqueness of alcoholics is not greatly aided by the seven items that were common to all three scales. These seven items are: "I have not lived the right kind of life" (True), "I go to church almost every week" (False), "I know who is responsible for most of my troubles" (True), "I have used alcohol excessively" (True), "I have never been in trouble with the law" (False), "The only miracles I know of are simply tricks that people play on one another" (False), and "I have used alcohol moderately or not at all (False). Note that we have already encountered the first, fourth, and fifth in the analysis of Scale 4 and the seventh item is merely the negative of the fourth.

Despite the vast differences in the item composition of these scales, each scale was reported by its authors to have succeeded at least to some degree in differentiating alcoholics from normals on cross-validation. To determine whether the three scales were tapping something unique to alcoholics, MacAndrew and Geertsma (1964) compared the scores of 300 male outpatient alcoholics on all three scales with the scores of 300 nonalcoholics and nondrug-abusing male psychiatric outpatients. The resulting point-biserial correlations were .22 for the Hampton scale, .34 for the Holmes scale, and .33 for the Hoyt–Sedlacek scale. When the two items that inquire directly about alcohol consumption were removed, these modest correlations were reduced to .17, .22, and .22, respectively. Removing all seven of the common items resulted in correlations of .13 for the remaining 118 items on the Hampton scale, .12 for the remaining 52 items on the Holmes scale, and .13 for the remaining 61 items on the Hoyt–Sedlacek scale. On the basis of these findings, MacAndrew and Geertsma (1964) concluded that the three scales did not measure alcoholism in any primary sense and thus they had little if any value for most clinical purposes. Working independently, Rotman and Vestre (1964) reached a similar conclusion by analyzing the scores of male alcoholic and psychiatric inpatients.

This conclusion has been challenged by Cox (1979) and by Rosenberg (1972) on the grounds that the correlations were statistically significant. These opposing appraisals nicely exemplify two approaches to the meaning of such significance: one informed by the dictum that "a difference that doesn't make a difference isn't a difference," the other by a rather single-minded concern for statistical significance. Cronbach (1970, p. 543) doubtless had the potential vacuity of the latter approach to significance in mind when he reminded us that, "Given enough cases, 'highly significant' differences can be established with instruments of no practical value."

One more observation must be made before leaving these data. Much has been said—and properly—against the purely rational or armchair approach to item selection—an approach in which items are generated on the basis of their seemingly obvious commonsensical or theoretical relationship to the criterion. Nevertheless, when the members of the two patient groups were scored solely on the two face-valid alcohol useage items, an r_{pb} of .80 was obtained. The moral here, of course, is that if the researcher's concern is only to detect persons who drink too much, the most efficient procedure is simply to ask.

If so little that differentiates alcoholics from normals differentiates them from other psychiatric outpatients as well, we may ask, Are alcoholics simply neurotics who also drink too much? More than a few psychologists, psychiatrists, and psychoanalysts contend that they are. To restate the question in a slightly different way, Is alcoholics' excessive use of alcohol a symptom of or a reaction to a disease process (psychiatrically conceived) but not a disease per se? To evaluate this possibility, MacAndrew (1965) compared the MMPI item responses of 200 adult male alcoholic outpatients with the MMPI item responses of 200 adult male psychiatric outpatients whose clinical files contained no indication of either alcohol or drug abuse. The presumption was that, if these two classes of psychiatric outpatients were similar save for their differential recourse to alcohol, it should be virtually impossible to discriminate between them. In fact, fifty-one items were found to differentiate between the two groups at the .01 level. After removing the two alcohol usage items, the remaining forty-nine items (which came to be called the MAC Scale) proved quite effective in differentiating between the two groups ($t = 18.62$; $p < .001$). This scale has now been cross-validated on three paired samples of male outpatients similar to those on whom the scale was constructed (Lachar and others, 1976; MacAndrew, 1965; Rhodes, 1969), and its discriminant capability has proven to be quite stable: $t = 23.28$, $p < .001$, for the combined cross-validation samples of 365 alcoholics versus 401 psychiatric outpatients (data summarized by MacAndrew, 1981b). In twenty-five additional published cross-validation samples of male alcoholics (data summarized by MacAndrew, 1981b), both the means and, when reported, the standard deviations and "detection rates" have been found to be almost identical to the values provided by the scale's original alcoholic standardization sample. Such findings clearly contradict the proposition that the majority of male alcoholics are simply neurotics who also drink too much.

The MAC Scale is not unique to alcoholism, however. Both MAC Scale means and, when reported, standard deviations and detection rates of six independently obtained samples of male drug abusers proved to be statistically indistinguishable from those of male alcoholics (data summarized by MacAndrew, 1981b). Furthermore, Rathus and others (1980), who used an abbreviated version of the MAC Scale on large samples of both male and female suburban high school students, found that high scores were related to self-reports not only of alcohol and drug usage but also of theft, violence, and property destruction. In a similar vein, Ruff and others (1975) found that the scores of small samples of adult male alcoholic inpatients and of nonalcoholic criminally charged patients from a forensic unit of the same hospital were statistically indistinguishable.

The final blow to the proposition that a scale to differentiate alcoholics from the rest of humankind can be contructed from the MMPI item pool was provided by Conley and Kammeier (1980). They found that only seven of the MMPI's 550 items differentiated ($p < .05$) their relatively large samples of mostly middle-class male and female alcoholics from their samples of male and female normals and neurotics on both derivational and cross-validational runs. What is more, two of the seven items referred directly to the nature of the individual's drinking practices, while two other items almost certainly referred to the phenomenon of alcoholic blackouts.

These findings from the scale approach provide scant support for the proposition that alcoholics are of a single piece, much less that they are uniquely so, and they provide no grounds whatsoever for supposing that the results of more sophisticated or more prodigious MMPI-focused efforts to develop a scale unique to alcoholism can demonstrate otherwise. While the quest for a single and unique alcoholic personality structure may continue on other fronts—Barnes (1979), for example, recently made a heroic but fundamentally unconvincing attempt to breathe new life into the flagging search—and while the presumption that such a structure exists will doubtless continue to operate on an ideological level, it is clear that past efforts have come to naught as far as the MMPI is concerned.

The Quest for a Taxonomy of Alcoholics

Even if alcoholics do not share a single or unique personality structure, it may be possible to order their personalities into a manageable number of subtypes. That is the premise of the profile approach. Here, too, MMPI-focused research efforts—now taxonomic in nature—began with what was already at hand: the MMPI standard scales. Specifically, the taxonomic enterprise began with classification codes built on the differential elevations of the standard clinical scales, most frequently with coding systems based on the most highly elevated pairs of these scales. Somewhat later, more complicated sets of mechanical decision rules based on the diverse relationships among subjects' scores on the several standard scales were used.

Recently, Schroeder and Piercy (1979) compared findings from four large samples of alcoholics ($N = 323$, 920, 1,009, and 2,570), in which subjects were categorized on the basis of the conventional two high-point coding systems. These authors, like many before them (see the summary of findings in Cox, 1979), found that Scale 2 (Depression) and Scale 4 (Psychopathic Deviate) were the ones most often elevated. However, the average percentage of 2–4 and 4–2 profiles in these four samples of alcoholics was found to be only 16.5 percent. "Most striking," these authors concluded (Schroeder and

Piercy, 1979, p. 662), "was the large number of [different] two-point code pairs that appeared in all [four] of the alcoholic samples." The search for a manageable number of discrete alcoholic subtypes by recourse to the more complexly structured sets of mechanical decision rules assembled by Gilberstadt and Ducker (1965) and by Marks and Seeman (1963) proved no more rewarding. Fowler and Coyle (1968), for example, found that these two sets of decision rules succeeded in classifying only 27 percent and 28 percent, respectively, of their combined sample of 231 male and 69 female outpatient alcoholics and that together these two sets of decision rules classified only 44 percent of their total sample.

If we consider such findings as these in conjunction with the findings reported from the scale approach, with findings that the average MMPI profiles of samples of alcoholics drawn from different treatment facilities are sometimes quite different, and with Rosen's (1960) finding that, although the average MMPI profile of his sample of alcoholics did not differ from that of a sample of general psychiatric patients who were being treated at the same outpatient facility, it did differ from the profiles of alcoholic samples drawn from other treatment facilities, we realize quite clearly that the presumption of a single homogeneous alcoholic personality cannot be sustained.

Faced with the limited taxonomic utility of such prepackaged sets of decision rules as those provided by Gilberstadt and Ducker (1965) and by Marks and Seeman (1963), the quest for a viable taxonomy of drinkers has become increasingly bootstrap in recent years. Following Gray (1973), we distinguish two general approaches to the construction of taxonomies: the approach of the splitter, whose quest is for a set of precise, relatively specific, and exhaustive categories, and the approach of the joiner, whose quest is for a small number of broad general categories. To help us understand this distinction, Gray suggests that, within the domain of factor analysis, Cattell, Guilford, and Thurstone can be placed among the splitters, while Eysenck, Spearman, and Vernon must be located among the joiners. The distinction is one of both general theoretical predilection and research strategy.

For those who have used the MMPI, the work of the splitters has typically involved application of one or another form of cluster or factor analysis to alcoholics' scores on the standard MMPI scales, to which a few MMPI special scales have sometimes been added. Since this approach—exemplified in the studies of Bean and Karasievich (1975), Goldstein and Linden (1969), Nerviano and others (1980), Skinner and others (1974), and Whitelock and others (1971)—is covered in Chapter Six of this volume, I shall limit my discussion to a taxonomy constructed by the joiner's strategy.

Since the MAC Scale was instrumental in specification of the typology, I shall begin by enumerating some findings obtained from work with this scale: In sixteen cross-validation samples of male alcoholics (data summarized by MacAndrew, 1981b), the percentage of MAC Scale true positives averaged approximately 85 percent (range: 79 percent to 97.5 percent). Similar percentages of true positives were reported (data summarized by MacAndrew, 1971b) for four samples of male drug abusers (range: 85 percent to 100 percent). Further, the MMPI item response rates of a sample of male alcoholic false negatives were found to be indistinguishable from those of a sample of male psychiatric outpatient true negatives who were not substance abusers (MacAndrew, 1979a), which suggests that a minority of male alcoholics are in fact neurotics who also drink too much. Moreover, the average MAC Scale scores of samples of young male alcohol offenders ($N = 79$; mean age $= 18.8 \pm 1.48$) and of nonsubstance-abusing young male psychiatric outpatients ($N = 48$; mean age $= 19.2 \pm 1.42$) were found to be indistinguishable from MAC Scale scores of samples of adult male counterparts (MacAndrew, 1981b). Finally, data of several sorts (summarized by MacAndrew, 1981b) indicate that the MAC Scale taps a broad, bipolar orientation to the world that can be characterized in terms either of the world's potentially rewarding character or of its potentially punishing character.

From these findings, I conclude (at a level of first approximation) that there exist—either as tendencies or full-blown—at least two fundamentally different, age-independent characterological types with samples of male alcoholics and drug abusers (MacAndrew, 1979a, 1980, 1981b). Primary alcoholics are those whose orientation to the world is in terms of its potentially rewarding character—the reward-seeking orientation of the majority of alcoholics on whom MAC Scale data have been published. Secondary or reactive alcoholics are those whose orientation to the world is in terms of its potentially punishing character—the punishment-avoidance orientation of the minority of alcoholics in such samples.

I have also found (MacAndrew, 1981a) that, compared to putatively normal adult males, male alcoholics of both character orientations (as well as nonsubstance-abusing male psychiatric outpatients) score very high on criterion group-derived and factorially pure scales of emotional tension and depression. Since these scales are both highly intercorrelated and approximately orthogonal to the MAC Scale, clearly it is not having different levels of tension, depression, or both that distinguishes primary from secondary alcoholics. Rather, it is their reaction to tension and depression that distinguishes them. Primary alcoholics drink and respond both actively and impulsively (drunken acting out), while secondary alcoholics appear to drink in the service of palliation. In this connection, it is instructive to note that, while the scores of young male nonsubstance-abusing psychiatric outpatients ($N = 48$; mean age $= 19.2 \pm 1.42$ years) are indistinguishable from those of their adult counterparts on these two scales, the scores of young male alcohol offenders ($N = 91$; mean age $= 18.9 \pm 1.45$ years) are indistinguishable from those of putatively normal male college students and very much lower than those of their adult counterparts (MacAndrew, 1982). This finding suggests that, for primary alcoholics, emotional tension and depression make their appearance not before (as has been conventionally supposed for alcoholics in general) but only at some point after young male offenders' use of alcohol has begun to cause problems.

Although correlates of the two alcoholic types are only now beginning to be reported, there is evidence that primary alcoholics tend to begin to drink heavily at an earlier age and that they are more likely to report having experienced symptoms of minimal brain dysfunction in childhood than secondary alcoholics are (Tarter and others, 1977). There is suggestive evidence, too, that suicidal concerns and acts are more likely to occur in nonalcoholic persons whose character orientation is similar to that of the secondary (reactive) alcoholic (Leonard, 1977).

Much remains to be done to clarify the relevance of drinkers' locations in the two-space schema created by these two orthogonal dimensions of reward-seeking versus punishment avoidance and high versus low tension and depression. In what ways, for instance, do drinkers of the two character orientations differentially avail themselves of the time-out option (MacAndrew and Edgerton, 1969), which in our society accompanies the status of being-in-the-world-drunk? Might the two types benefit differently from the current array of treatment modalities and services? Do they contribute differentially to such family problems as incest, child battering, and wife beating, in which drunkenness of the transgressor is so frequently implicated? Are the two types differently involved in the perpetration of other categories of crime? What about the drunk driver? Does one of the two types contribute disproportionately to the alcohol-implicated carnage on our nation's highways?

It should be evident from the nature of these questions that I am in the camp of those who hold that, if we are ever to begin to solve the alcohol problem, the first thing we must do is to unpackage it. Progress will come not from the discovery of a key to alcoholism but only from piecemeal analyses of the many specific and often mundane problems to which the consumption of alcohol is either known or presumed to give rise.

As for the criterion problem to which the disease formulation gave rise, it has been finessed by the recognition that the sundry specific problems to which the consumption of alcohol either directly or indirectly gives rise stand in sublime independence of whether the person who causes the problem in any concrete case has or has not been accorded the diagnosis of alcoholism. Furthermore, since the treatment of such alcohol-engendered conditions as hepatic liver would be treated no differently whether the sufferer was truly an alcoholic or merely a heavy drinker, I can conceive of no procedural reason why this unpackaging process ought to be limited solely to difficulties that we term *social*.

Conclusions

The mass of findings generated by analyses of alcoholics' responses to the MMPI provides no support for the notion that such persons share a common—much less, a unique—personality structure, nor is there any reason to suppose that future efforts will succeed in this regard where past efforts have failed. Thus, I suggested that the development of a viable taxonomy of drinkers constitutes the only reasonable focus for future research. Such taxonomic efforts can assume the strategy either of the splitter or of the joiner. I concluded by presenting an MMPI-derived exemplification of the second strategy.

References

Atsaides, J. P., Neuringer, C., and Davis, K. L. "Development of an Institutionalized Chronic Alcoholic Scale." *Journal of Consulting and Clinical Psychology,* 1977, *45,* 609–611.

Barnes, G. E. "The Alcoholic Personality: A Reanalysis of the Literature." *Journal of Studies on Alcohol,* 1979, *40,* 571–634.

Bean, K. L., and Karasievich, G. O. "Psychological Test Results at Three Stages of Inpatient Alcoholism Treatment." *Journal of Studies on Alcohol,* 1975, *36,* 838–852.

Button, A. D. "A Study of Alcoholic with the MMPI." *Quarterly Journal of Studies on Alcohol,* 1956, *17,* 263–281.

Conley, J. J., and Kammeier, M .L. "Alcoholism-Related Content in the MMPI: Item Analysis of Alcoholics Versus Normal and General Psychiatric Populations." In M. Gallanter (Ed.), *Currents in Alcoholism.* Vol. 7: *Recent Advances in Research and Treatment.* New York: Grune & Stratton, 1980.

Cox, W. M. "The Alcoholic's Personality: A Review of the Evidence." In B. A. Maher (Ed.), *Progress in Experimental Personality Research.* Vol. 9. New York: Academic Press, 1979.

Cronbach, L. J. *Essentials of Psychological Testing.* (3rd ed.) New York: Harper & Row, 1970.

Fowler, R. D., and Coyle, F. A. "A Comparison of Two MMPI Actuarial Systems Used in Classifying an Alcoholic Outpatient Population." *Journal of Clinical Psychology,* 1968, *24,* 434–435.

Gilberstadt, H., and Ducker, J. *Handbook for Clinical and Actuarial MMPI Interpretation.* Philadelphia: Saunders, 1965.

Goldstein, S. G., and Linden, J. D. "Multivariate Classification of Alcoholics by Means of the MMPI." *Journal of Abnormal Psychology,* 1969, *74,* 661–669.

Gray, J. A. "Causal Theories of Personality and How to Test Them." In J. R. Royce, (Ed.), *Multivariate Analysis and Psychological Theory.* New York: Academic Press, 1973.

Hampton, P. J. "The Development of a Personality Questionnaire for Drinkers." *Genetic Psychology Monographs,* 1953, *48,* 55–115.

Hathaway, S. R. "Forewords" to the First and Second Editions. In W. G. Dahlstrom, G. S. Welsh, and L. E. Dahlstrom, *An MMPI Handbook.* Vol. 1: *Clinical Interpretation.* (Rev. ed.) Minneapolis: University of Minnesota Press, 1972.

Holmes, W. O. "The Development of an Empirical MMPI Scale for Alcoholism." Unpublished master's thesis, San Jose State College, 1953.

Hoyt, D. P., and Sedlacek, G. M. "Differentiating Alcoholics from Normals and Abnormals with the MMPI." *Journal of Clinical Psychology,* 1958, *14,* 69–74.

Keller, M. "The Oddities of Alcoholics." *Quarterly Journal of Studies on Alcohol,* 1972, *33,* 1147–1148.

Lachar, D., Berman, W., Grisell, J. L., and Schoof, K. "The MacAndrew Alcoholism Scale as a General Measure of Substance Misuse." *Journal of Studies on Alcohol,* 1976, *37,* 1609–1615.

Leonard, C. V. "The MMPI as a Suicide Predictor." *Journal of Consulting and Clinical Psychology,* 1977, *45,* 367–377.

MacAndrew, C. "The Differentiation of Male Alcoholic Outpatients from Nonalcoholic Psychiatric Outpatients by Means of the MMPI." *Quarterly Journal of Studies on Alcohol,* 1965, *26,* 238–246.

MacAndrew, C. "On the Notion That Certain Persons Who Are Given to Frequent Drunkenness Suffer from a Disease Called Alcoholism." In S. C. Plog and R. B. Edgerton (Eds.), *Changing Perspectives in Mental Illness.* New York: Holt, Rinehart and Winston, 1969.

MacAndrew, C. "Women Alcoholics' Responses to Scale 4 of the MMPI." *Journal of Studies on Alcohol,* 1978, *39,* 1841–1854.

MacAndrew, C. "Evidence for the Presence of Two Fundamentally Different, Age-Independent Characterological Types Within Unselected Runs of Male Alcohol and Drug Abusers." *American Journal of Drug and Alcohol Abuse,* 1979a, *6,* 207–221.

MacAndrew, C. "On the Possibility of the Psychometric Detection of Persons Who Are Prone to the Abuse of Alcohol and Other Substances." *Addictive Behaviors,* 1979b, *4,* 11–20.

MacAndrew, C. "Male Alcoholics, Secondary Psychopathy, and Eysenck's Theory of Personality." *Personality and Individual Differences,* 1980, *1,* 151–160.

MacAndrew, C. "Similarities in the Self-Depictions of Men Alcoholics and Psychiatric Outpatients: An Examination of Eysenck's Dimension of Emotionality." *Journal of Studies on Alcohol,* 1981a, *42,* 421–431.

MacAndrew, C. "What the MAC Scale Tells Us about Men Alcoholics: An Interpretive Review." *Journal of Studies on Alcohol,* 1981b, *42,* 604–625.

MacAndrew, C. "An Examination of the Relevance of the Individual Differences (A-Trait) Formulation of the Tension Reduction Theory to the Etiology of Alcohol Abuse in Young Males." *Addictive Behaviors,* 1982, *7,* 39–45.

MacAndrew, C., and Edgerton, R. B. *Drunken Comportment: A Social Explanation.* Chicago: Aldine, 1969.

MacAndrew, C., and Geertsma, R. H. "An Analysis of Responses of Alcoholics to Scale 4 of the MMPI." *Quarterly Journal of Studies on Alcohol,* 1963, *24,* 23–38.

MacAndrew, C., and Geertsma, R. H. "A Critique of Alcoholism Scales Derived from the MMPI." *Quarterly Journal of Studies on Alcohol,* 1964, *25,* 68–76.

Marks, P. A., and Seeman, W. *Actuarial Description of Abnormal Personality: An Atlas for Use with the MMPI.* Baltimore: Williams and Wilkins, 1963.

Miller, W. R. "Alcoholism Scales and Objective Assessment Methods: A Review." *Psychological Bulletin,* 1976, *83,* 649–674.

Nerviano, V. J., McCarty, D., and McCarty, S. M. "MMPI Profile Patterns of Men Alcoholics in Two Contrasting Settings." *Journal of Studies on Alcohol,* 1980, *41,* 1143–1152.

Rathus, S. A., Fox, J. A., and Ortins, J. B. "The MacAndrew Scale as a Measure of Substance Abuse and Delinquency Among Adolescents." *Journal of Clinical Psychology,* 1980, *36,* 579–583.

Rhodes, R. J. "The MacAndrew Alcoholism Scale: A Replication." *Journal of Clinical Psychology,* 1969, *25,* 189–191.

Rich, C. C., and Davis, H. G. "Concurrent Validity of MMPI Alcoholism Scales." *Journal of Clinical Psychology,* 1969, *25,* 425–426.

Rosen, A. C. "A Comparative Study of Alcoholic and Psychiatric Patients with the MMPI." *Quarterly Journal of Studies on Alcohol,* 1960, *21,* 253–266.

Rosenberg, N. "MMPI Alcoholism Scales." *Journal of Clinical Psychology,* 1972, *28,* 515–522.

Rotman, S. R., and Vestre, N. D. "The Use of the MMPI in Identifying Problem Drinkers Among Psychiatric Hospital Admissions." *Journal of Clinical Psychology,* 1964, *20,* 526–530.

Ruff, C. F., Ayes, J., and Templer, D. I. "Alocholics' and Criminals' Similarity of Scores on the MacAndrew Alcoholism Scale." *Psychological Reports,* 1975, *36,* 921–922.

Schroeder, D. J., and Piercy, D. C. "A Comparison of MMPI Two-Point Codes in Four Alcoholism Treatment Facilities." *Journal of Clinical Psychology,* 1979, *35,* 656–663.

Seeley, J. R. "Alcoholism Is a Disease: Implications for Social Policy." In D. J. Pittman and C. R. Snyder (Eds.), *Society, Culture, and Drinking Patterns.* New York: Wiley, 1962.

Skinner, H. A., Jackson, D. N., and Hoffmann, H. "Alcoholic Personality Types: Identification and Correlates." *Journal of Abnormal Psychology,* 1974, *83,* 658–666.

Tarter, R. E., McBride, H., Buonpane, N., and Schneider, D. U. "Differentiation of Alcoholics: Childhood History of Minimal Brain Dysfunction, Family History, and Drinking Pattern." *Archives of General Psychiatry,* 1977, *34,* 761–768.

Whitelock, P. R., Overall, J. E., and Patrick, J. H. "Personality Patterns and Alcohol Abuse in a State Hospital Population." *Journal of Abnormal Psychology,* 1971, *78,* 9–16.

Craig MacAndrew is professor of psychology at the University of California, Irvine. He has engaged in research on alcohol and alcoholism for many years.

Are patterns of excessive alcohol consumption associated with different syndromes of measured psychopathology and neuropsychological dysfunction?

Differential Personality Inventory Types Among Alcoholics

Douglas N. Jackson

"Research, treatment, and prevention of the various species of alcoholism are affected not only by the acceptance or rejection of the disease conception but also by the formulation of the nature of such an illness." With these words, Jellinek (1960, p. 158) highlighted the implications that particular conceptions of alcoholism have for prevention and treatment. Jellinek recognized the complex interplay between economic, social, and moral conceptions on the one hand and psychological, physiological, and medical conceptions on the other that created discrete species of alcoholics, not a single homogeneous set of behaviors characterizing excessive alcohol intake. In this chapter, I present evidence bearing on a different but related issue—that different types of psychopathology are associated with severe alcoholism. Just as evidence supports the idea that there is more than one species of symptomatic alcoholism, I offer evidence that there is more than one alcoholic personality type.

In introducing the question of alcoholic personalities, it is useful to distinguish between the personality existing prior to the onset of major alcoholic addiction (the topic of the chapter by Cox and others in this volume) and the personality and psychopathology manifesting itself partly as a function of the physiological, psychological, and social consequences of drinking. Although this is an easy conceptual distinction, it is difficult in practice (as we saw in the chapter by Cox and others) because it is rare that alcoholics are identified for

W. M. Cox (Ed.). *Identifying and Measuring Alcoholic Personality Characteristics.* New Directions for Methodology of Social and Behavioral Science, no. 16. San Francisco: Jossey-Bass, June 1983.

study prior to the time when the consequences of alcohol are observed. With only a few exceptions, alcoholics are studied after the disease and degenerative processes have taken some toll. Classification studies of the psychopathology of alcoholics thus represent systematic attempts to study the psychological consequences of drinking as much as or more than they do the personality structure independent of processes linked to alcohol addicition. As Loper and Cox point out, to distinguish these two issues requires large-scale longitudinal research using the general population.

There are at least three important reasons for studying the multivariate classification of psychopathology associated with alcoholism, even if the psychopathology is regarded as a result of the alcoholic addiction process: First, alcoholism is not a discrete homogeneous state but progressive (Jellinek, 1946). Studies over time of the unfolding patterns of causal links between alcoholism and psychopathology depend on accurate classification of psychopathology as well as on assessment of alcoholism. Second, treatment research should not only address the nature of the symptomatic alcoholism, it should also evaluate efficacy in relation to types of associated psychopathology. It is possible that treatment of alcoholism is differentially effective as a function of the type of associated psychopathology. Third, when personality changes occur in association with alcoholism, some are likely to prove irreversible and exist on their own apart from the symptomatic drinking. The identification of the processes leading to psychopathology deserve study and depend on accurate classification.

There are two major traditions in psychological thinking about the classification of deviant behavior: that based on a dimensional framework and that tied to conceptions of types or diagnostic categories. Many authors have noted the limitations of each tradition when it is applied to persons who abuse alcohol. Since both symptomatic drinking and its consequences vary widely in their manifestations, many clinicians and investigators have despaired of defining a single dimension of alcoholism. Similarly, while serious work has sometimes highlighted the diversity of persons who suffer from alcohol abuse, both informal and diagnostic language continue to use the words *alcoholic* and *alcoholism* in contexts where the intent (and effect) is to communicate more than excessive drinking, and to imply a distinctive and homogeneous set of personality characteristics and psychopathological behaviors. We need to examine critically the basis for this implicit theorizing, because it has serious consequences both for scientific thinking about problems concerning alcohol and for treatment.

This chapter bears four important messages about the classification of behavior and psychopathology associated with alcohol abuse. First, close attention needs to be paid to the nature of the constructs of psychopathology on which classification is based. Second, conceptions that combine dimensional, measurement approaches with multivariate classification are more productive than conceptions based on simple orderings or categories. Third, developmental, physiological, and social influences affect any classification system. Finally, the scope of efforts to understand the basis for clustering alcoholics needs to be expanded.

The studies described in this chapter illustrate these points. The first two studies were designed to identify consistent, replicated personality types among alcoholic patients with the Differential Personality Inventory (DPI). The third, a recent study using the Minnesota Multiphasic Personality Inventory (MMPI), illustrates the implications of personality-derived profiles for the understanding of drinking history and neuropsychological deficits. Finally, a critique of present classificatory efforts is combined with a forward-looking perspective on suggestions for further research in this area.

The Differential Personality Inventory (Jackson and Messick, 1983) is a questionnaire developed from the construct-oriented strategy of test construction (Jackson, 1971; Wiggins, 1973). Designed to measure twenty-eight measures of psychopathology, this 432-item inventory spans a broad array of personality dimensions, ranging from Perceptual Distortion and Feelings of Unreality to Defensiveness and Shallow Affect. In the test development program, considerable attention was devoted to defining independent constructs of psychopathology, preparing large pools of items bearing both theoretical and empirical links to the underlying construct, suppressing response styles, and fostering convergent and discriminant validity as well as substantive generalizability and scale independence. Partington and Johnson (1969) reported a median internal consistency reliability of .80 for the subset of the scales that they used. Jackson and Carlson (1973) reported a set of external validity coefficients using roommate ratings, all significant at the .001 level, for a shorter version of fifteen scales. The following is a list of scale names and sample items for seventeen of the twenty-seven scales.

Desirability	I liked my school principal and most of my teachers.
Defensiveness	I have never cheated in any matter.
Cynicism	There is no such thing as an honest lawyer.
Hostility	I believe that physical violence is often justified.
Rebelliousness	I hate to be told what to do.
Socially Deviant Attitudes	I believe in grabbing everything I can get in this world.
Health Concern	I worry a great deal about my health.
Headache Proneness	I frequently get headaches.
Hypochondriasis	The lining of my stomach is too thin.
Shallow Affect	It is very hard for me to get excited over anything.
Infrequency	I have never had more than two teeth.
Neurotic Disorganization	I often cannot make up my mind.
Irritability	Often, people say things that seem to "grate" on my nerves.

Impulsivity	I usually act upon the first thought that comes into my head.
Familial Discord	I fight a lot with my family.
Somatic Complaints	I often have an upset stomach.
Depression	Most things that I do turn out to be failures.

Note: Items copyrighted 1976 by Douglas N. Jackson and Samuel Messick. All rights reserved.

In my view, explicit constructs of psychopathology have a number of advantages over scales defined empirically by virtue of the correlation of their items with an external criterion, both in classification research and elsewhere. If such scales are properly constructed, they allow relatively homogeneous sets of behavior to be attributed to the respondent—in short, they are interpretable. They also have a certain internal coherence, in that they do not depend on some unstated rule for an administrative decision, as they do when criterion diagnostic groups are used to construct scales. In addition, such scales fit well with classical conceptions of psychometric theory, since they provide a theoretical basis for suppressing sources of response bias and other nuisance or contaminating variables. Moreover, low scores from scales based on explicit constructs permit inferences about the behavior of individuals more than empirically derived scales do. Finally, empirical studies have demonstrated that scales based on defined constructs are consistently more valid than empirically derived scales.

Our intent in selecting scales for inclusion in the DPI was to sample broadly from the domain of psychopathology, including not only dysfunctions of cognition (Perceptual Distortion, Broodiness, and Ideas of Persecution) and dysfunctions of mood and affect (Depression, Mood Fluctuation, Shallow Affect) but also disorders of attitude and character development (Socially Deviant Attitudes, Cynicism, Rebelliousness, Hostility) and disorders involving health preoccupation and somatization (Somatic Complaints, Headache Proneness, Hypochondriasis, and Health Concern). Although it is probably not possible to devise a scale that reflects a single dimension of neuroticism, scales reflecting Panic Reaction, Insomnia, Defensiveness, and Neurotic Disorganization can capture facets of neuroticism. I contend that all these scales contribute to an understanding of persons who abuse alcohol, but none in itself is sufficient to provide more than a grossly abbreviated picture of a disordered personality. However, if such scales are combined in a profile, they can tell us much about psychopathology, including cognitive, affective, characterological, and interpersonal facets.

A Multivariate Dimensional Approach to Classification of Psychopathology

The term *alcoholic* is a label that has its origins in the sociology of labelling (Paquin and Jackson, 1981). It designates persons who have little more in common than their having been identified as individuals whose behavior has been a nuisance (or worse) for reasons ascribed to drinking. It is very much of a seven-league jump from the label to the idea that such persons necessarily share a single, homogeneous set of personality characteristics that distinguish them both from the general population and from other deviant groups. Of course, the traditional approach, which limits comparisons between persons designated as alcoholics and others to examination of mean differences, is based on the assumption that alcoholics share a set of characteristics. This assumption usually precludes identification of subtypes within the alcoholic population. For example, if two types equally deviant in opposite directions were averaged, they might show little or no discrepancy in personality scale scores when compared with a sample from the general population, although each type might be quite distinctly pathological. Average scores of distinct types would be particularly misleading in treatment studies, where changes could go unrecognized if they occurred in opposite and compensating directions (Partington and Johnson, 1969).

Others have implied a similar view in classification studies. In one pioneering study, Goldstein and Linden (1969) applied Lorr's method of multivariate clustering to MMPI profile data and identified four subgroups, which were later cross-replicated. Since that time, sixteen more classification studies using the MMPI have come to my attention. Most of these studies are discussed in the careful review by Morey and Blashfield (1981). These studies used a variety of indexes of profile similarity (usually a correlational or distance measure) and a variety of clustering techniques.

The Partington and Johnson Study. In the same year that the Goldstein–Linden study was published, Partington and Johnson (1969) reported their findings. The subjects, 186 male patients comprising first admissions to an outpatient clinic (the Alcohol and Drug Addiction Research Foundation of Ontario), ranged in age between twenty-three and fifty-eight and reported an average 8.2 years of problem drinking. Subjects were administered an experimental form of eighteen Differential Personality Inventory scales (Jackson and Messick, 1976), a medical examination, intelligence tests, and case history interviews, and they were rated by a psychiatrist on a number of dimensions, including motivation for treatment, degree of self-understanding, and prognosis. A preliminary components analysis reduced the eighteen-scale DPI profile to four more general dimensions—Stylistic Responding, Antisocial Tendencies, Neuroticism, and Thought Disorder. (For example, Socially Deviant Attitudes, Hostility, Cynicism, and Rebelliousness were reduced to a single dimension, Antisocial Tendencies.) Each profile was then classified using multivariate procedures. Five replicated types were identified. Each showed a different pattern of DPI responding as well as a unique structure of drinking, demographic, clinical, and social patterns, which differed significantly among themselves. These types are of considerable interest.

Type I (20 percent of the sample) was characterized on the DPI by low defensiveness and high antisocial and thought disturbance tendencies. Type I patients were insensitive to the interpretation that others placed on their behavior and manifested impulsivity, rebelliousness and interpersonal conflict, labile emotions, and disorganization of thinking. In criterion behavior, such persons tended to be young, showed an unstable employment record, and reported serious consequences of drinking. Independent psychiatric ratings were consistent with the DPI—social instability, chronic depression and anxiety, aggression and antisocial tendencies, and lack of motivation for treatment coupled with poor prognosis.

Type II patients comprised 19 percent of the total sample. Their profile showed moderately low antisocial and moderately high thought disturbance components. Results suggested that these patients sometimes lose emotional and cognitive control. Their demographic data indicated high verbal intelligence, poor marital status, and relatively mild drinking problems compared with those of the other types. The drinking practices and record of abstinence of this type appeared to be the most favorable of all the types. The psychiatrist rated Type II patients as very interested in the treatment process and as having great insight into their problems and a good prognosis.

The other types were equally distinct. Type III patients (10 percent) were older, less intelligent, and more neurotic, with poor motivation for abstinence. Type IV patients (23 percent) were more defensive and showed fewer antisocial tendencies than the members of any other group. Type V patients (28 percent) were the heaviest and most frequent drinkers, but otherwise they were the best adjusted of the patients studied.

The Skinner, Jackson, and Hoffmann Study. The study by Skinner, Jackson, and Hoffmann (1974) refined a classification procedure developed by Jackson and Williams (1975) to identify recurring profile types in the DPI records of 282 patients admitted to a psychiatric hospital that specialized in treatment of persons suffering from severe symptoms of alcohol abuse. The classification procedure that these authors employed, modal profile analysis, involved dividing the 282 patients into three groups of 94 patients each so that analysis of the twenty-eight-scale DPI profiles could be replicated and confirmed on distinct samples. The analysis attempted to classify patients into clusters, such that the DPI profiles within each cluster had similar shapes. These clusters were projected onto axes that were rotated so that a single cluster, representing a particular profile type, was salient on the axis. Often, clusters were bipolar, so that a cluster sharing an opposite profile type was represented on the alternative pole of the typal dimension. Replication was considered important, because it adds to the confidence placed on the identification of profile types. The fact that profiles appear in three randomly assigned samples considerably improves the chances that they represent stable personality types.

Analysis revealed that sixteen clusters could be represented in an eight-dimensional space, with one of the clusters salient on each pole of the eight typal dimensions. An illustration of Dimensions I and II is shown in Figure 1. The DPI scale names salient for each of the profile types are indicated in Figure 1. Scale names listed adjacent to the positive poles of Dimensions I and II define the profile clusters with the respective positive projections, while scale names listed adjacent to the negative poles describe the negatively related clusters. (Scale names listed beside a given group centroid for a cluster are scales with high points on the corresponding modal profile, while scale names listed opposite are those with low points.) Figure 2 displays the contrast between two individuals, one scoring high and one scoring low with respect to typal Dimension I. These two profiles are virtual mirror images and provide concrete evidence of the error that lies in assuming that alcoholics necessarily manifest homogeneous patterns of psychopathology.

The variety of characteristic patterns of psychopathology is evident from an examination of the salient DPI scales for the sixteen clusters described

Figure 1. Group Centroids for Patients Classified to Common Types I and II

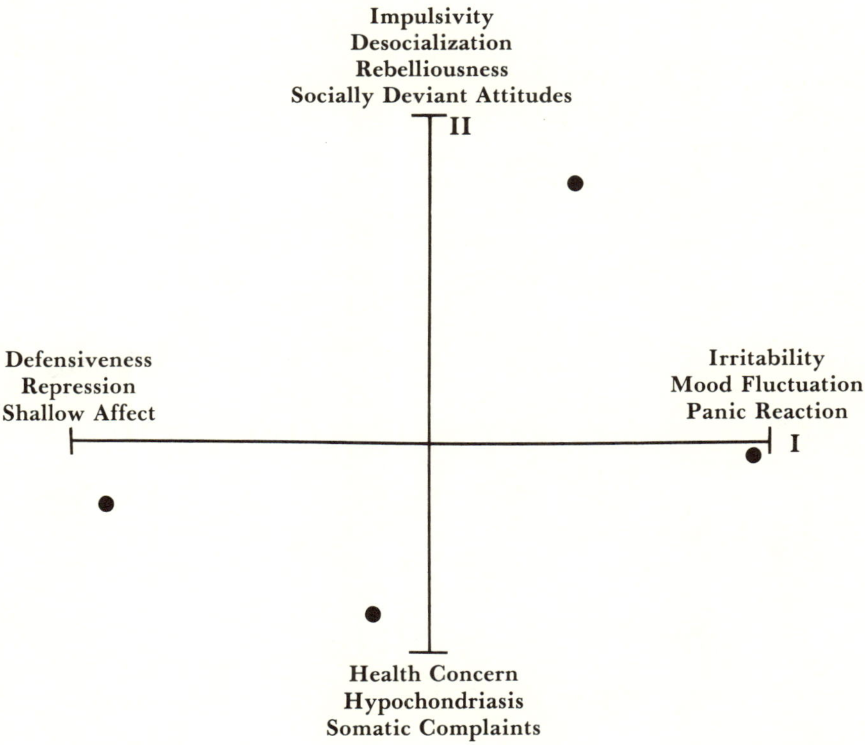

Note: The closed circles denote the respective group centroids of clusters defining opposite poles of the two dimensions. (Reprinted with permission from an article by Skinner, H. A., Jackson, D. N., and Hoffmann, H., 1974.)

Figure 2. Differential Personality Profiles of Two Patients Scoring at Opposite Poles of Typal Dimension I.

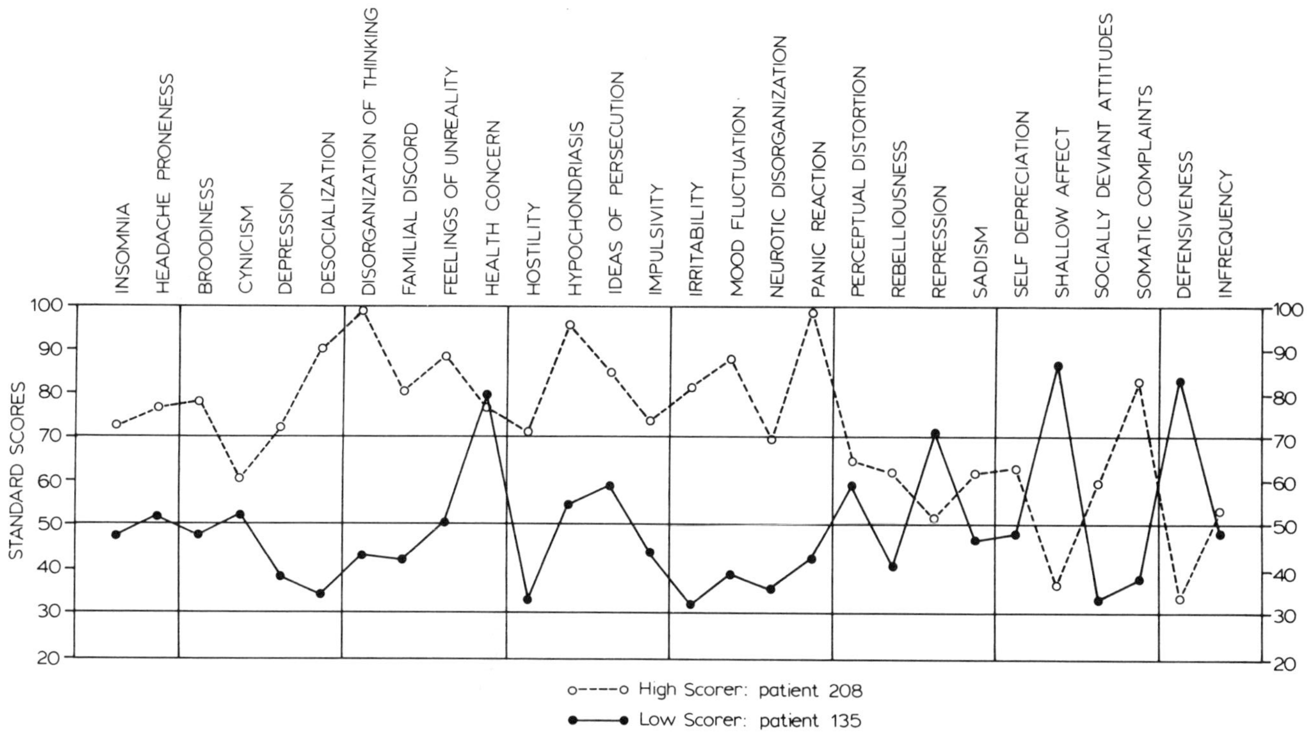

Table 1. Salient DPI Scales for Modal Profiles

Profile	Negative Pole	Positive Pole
I	Defensiveness, repression, shallow affect	Irritability, panic reaction, mood fluctuation
II	Health concern, hypochondriasis, somatic complaints	Rebelliousness, socially deviant attitudes, impulsivity, desocialization
III	Self-depreciation, cynicism, depression, health concern	Perceptual distortion, headache proneness, hostility, irritability
IV	Health concern, sadism, broodiness, ideas of persecution, hostility, familial discord, cynicism	Insomnia, self-depreciation, neurotic disorganization, defensiveness
V	Depression, rebelliousness, familial discord	Insomnia, sadism, health concern, neurotic disorganization
VI	Health concern, impulsivity, mood fluctuation, perceptual distortion	Hostility, sadism, family discord, desocialization, insomnia
VII	Cynicism, disorganization of thinking, perceptual distortion, rebelliousness	Insomnia, familial discord, health concern, mood fluctuation
VIII	Repression, irritability, cynicism, ideas of persecution, insomnia	Sadism, impulsivity, socially deviant attitudes, somatic complaints, hypochondriasis

in Table 1. Table 1 shows that patterns of high and low profile points can indeed be combined into cogent prototypes.

Finally, the eight DPI-based typal dimensions that replicated among the 282 alcoholic psychiatric patients were related to MMPI profile types identified in the systems of Goldstein and Linden (1969), Whitelock and others (1971), Lanyon (1968), and Marks and Seeman (1963). Relations with the four diagnostic systems provided strong evidence for pervasiveness of common type personality patterns among types in the general psychiatric population. For example, for Common Type I high scorers, who suffered from acute anxiety, the highest correlation was with Lanyon's (1968) alcoholic prototype. The highest correlation in the Marks and Seeman (1963) and Gilberstadt and Ducker (1965) systems was with their Code 2-7-4 types. According to Gilberstadt and Ducker (1965), the cardinal feature of this group is chronic alcoholism. After hospital admission, anxiety and depression are manifest symptoms, but prognosis is poor for effective treatment, since poor response is shown to therapeutic measures. In most instances, these authors state, the only benefit that hospitalization has to offer is a period of temporary drying out. In summary, the data suggest that Common Type I high scorers are similar to other classifications of patients showing personality patterns related to alcoholism.

In addition, several strong relationships were evident between low scorers on Common Type II (hypochondriacal preoccupation) and Lanyon's

(1968) hysteric, conversion reaction group, Marks and Seeman's (1963) Code 3–1, and Gilberstadt and Ducker's (1965) Code 1–3–2 patients diagnosed as psychoneurotics, conversion reaction with depression. Cardinal features include a hysteroid, passive-dependent character. Especially under stress, impulses that cause anxiety are converted into symptoms in organs or parts of the body. The positive pole of Common Type II (antisocial attitudes) had a moderate correlation with Lanyon's (1968) manic group.

In contrast to the distinct DPI profile for the sixteen individual types, the group DPI profile averaged over sixteen types was relatively flat, with significant elevations on only three scales (Health Concern, Ideas of Persecution, and Panic Reaction). A subsequent study (Skinner and others, 1976) revealed that the same types found among alcoholic patients could be identified in groups of prison inmates, psychiatric patients, and university students, although these groups differed both from alcoholics and from each other in the proportion of persons who could be classified in each set and in the average elevation of profiles within types. Furthermore, evidence reported by Reed and Jackson (1975) indicated that, when judges evaluated clinical prototypes, cases that bore a strong similarity to the modal profiles found in the earlier clustering study were judged more reliably. Indeed, group consensus judgments of the probability of behavior to be expected from cases prototypical of empirical types exceeded .98 (Reed and Jackson, 1975), a finding consistent with recent theorizing regarding conceptual prototypes (Canter and others, 1980).

Classification Studies Using the MMPI

A number of studies report diverse MMPI profile types among alcoholics (Donovan and others, 1978). Since these studies have been ably reviewed by Clopton (1978), Cox (1979), and Morey and Blashfield (1981), I shall only review the results of one recent comprehensive study that incorporated a number of desirable features. To 109 Norwegian males (mean age 39.8) who had a primary diagnosis of alcoholism, Løberg (1981) administered the MMPI and an extensive battery of other tests, including the Halstead–Reitan neuropsychological test battery and additional sensorimotor tests, the Wechsler Adult Intelligence Scale, and the Wechsler Memory Scale. Løberg also collected considerable data on alcohol intake and associated problems in a number of areas, including family problems and financial problems. Results indicated four reliable subtypes. Subtype A had a 4–2–5–3 profile, Subtype B had a 2–8–4 profile, Subtype C had a 2–8–7–4 profile, and Subtype D had an 8–2–4–7 profile. Different subtypes revealed distinctly different types of problems associated with drinking. Problems with friends and neighbors and belligerence characterized Subtype D. Subtype B reported the highest level of alcohol misuse, in contrast to Subtype A, which showed the least, but Subtype D reported a greater frequency of intoxication and blackouts. Important trends were evident in cognitive functioning. For example, subtypes were clearly separated in intelligence; Subtype D was the lowest, and Subtype A was the highest. Subtype D was also inferior on the Wechsler Memory Scale. Neuropsychological differences were evident as well. Relating these subtypes to previous research, Løberg identified Subtype A as a psychopathic personality, better educated, with higher intelligence, less neurological impairment, and less severe life disruption due to drinking than the other types. Subtype B exhibited a classical neurotic pattern, with psychological dependence reflecting an attempt to alleviate depression and anxiety and with little neuropsychological impairment. Subtype C corresponded to an actuarial description of pseudoneurotic or chronic undifferentiated schizophrenia, with evidence of greater involvement with the police and poorer intelligence, poorer memory, and poorer neuropsychological functioning that in Subtypes A and B. Subtype D corresponded to an actuarial description of paranoid type personality pattern disturbance, or paranoid-type schizophrenic reaction. Consistent with the psychotic-like MMPI profile, this subtype showed the greatest impairment as evidenced by early age of onset of drinking, conflicts with others, severe intoxication and blackouts, low intelligence, neuropsychological dysfunction, and poor memory. In fact, the characteristics of this group led Løberg to conjecture that prealcoholic central nervous system dysfunction or other etiological factors contributed to or interacted with alcoholism to produce the severe and deviant symptoms found.

If we compare Løberg's results with the results described earlier in this chapter, it becomes evident that Løberg's subtypes were both more general and less highly differentiated in terms of particular dimensions of psychopathology that the subtypes reported for the DPI. Although Løberg admits that his decision to analyze four MMPI profile types was somewhat arbitrary, we should recognize that the more global nature of the MMPI scales and their higher intercorrelations limit the number of types that can be derived from an evaluation of profile differences. Indeed, general personality types, such as those reported, may mask within-group differences that would be plain if the personality scales defining the groups were more differentiated. However, Løberg's study does illustrate how it is possible to integrate data from a personality questionnaire with data from a variety of other sources to derive a typology supporting the cross-situational generalizability of personality types linked to alcohol abuse.

Implications of Multivariate Classification for Research on Alcoholism

Changing Views of Measurement and Classification. Our views of the nature of alcoholism are changing, and fresh conceptual approaches to traditional problems and concomitant changes in techniques for measurement and classification are required (Skinner, 1981). We see five major shifts in focus:

First, the era in which a single discipline was omnipotent in providing an explanation for alcoholism is over. Recognition of the complexities of the determinants of alcoholism and of the need for interdisciplinary study is growing. Second, awareness of the multidimensional nature of causative agents is increasing. Third, the importance of the distinction between phenotype and genotype has been recognized. We need to go beyond simple observation to develop models that allow us to examine the structural relationships between underlying or latent variables. Fourth, measurement models that permit quantified, dimensional measurement, rather than simple classification, are being developed. Fifth, the search for viable links between classification systems and methods for treatment and intervention that take cost-benefit utilities into account is under way. These emerging trends point to the critical need both to develop more effective classification procedures and to make their results more useful to professionals charged with programs for alcoholism treatment and policy. A number of recommendations can be made regarding further research in this area. As others (Blashfield, 1980) have reported, there are a number of ways in which current research could be improved.

Directions for Future Classification Research in Alcohol Abuse. Current thinking about research methodology can be incorporated into studies that evaluate and classify the behavior of alcoholics. In the interests of brevity, I list these and a few of their implications. First, a number of levels of analysis should be incorporated into studies of alcoholism. As Jellinek (1960) noted, many authors pay lip service to the complex interplay of sociocultural, personological, and physiological processes, then limit their study to one facet of a single area. Broader studies and measurement models that do justice to the complex interplay just mentioned are needed. Second, the reliability of the classification system should be demonstrated routinely. Application of an efficient classification algorithm will usually yield apparent success, even with random numbers. Whether the same inferences can be drawn from another sample is not often reported, but such data are critical if we are to place confidence in the results. Third, the implications of applying different classification schemes and algorithms need to be recognized. Investigators sometimes choose a classification algorithm without a clear rationale, although their conception of the organization of the pathological behavior might have had a better fit with another model. Fourth, the nature of the constructs included in a classification framework needs careful attention. The blind empiricism of an earlier era has been criticized as unproductive (Blashfield, 1980). Furthermore, it is inefficient, and it is very unlikely to produce results relevant to important outcomes.

Awareness of the measurement problems of scores to be included in classification research needs to increase, and means for overcoming these problems need to be developed. Many classification studies are subject to criticism on a number of measurement-related grounds: for treating response bias and method variance as valid variance; for employing measures of unknown reliability; for using profiles whose constituent scores are highly intercorrelated and whose differential shapes are unreliable in analyzing profile similarity; for disregarding the construct validity of scores entering into classification; for mixing measurement models inappropriately, as when measures developed to predict a particular criterion are used as if they represented hypothetical constructs; and for illogical weighting of variables, often by inadvertence as in the use of variables showing markedly discrepant observed and true-score variances.

Moreover, the purposes of classification need to be related to the investigator's overall aims. It would be possible, for example, to develop measures of alcoholics based on their shoe size, forearm circumference, and similar measures, and classification based on such measures might prove reliable. But both its cross-domain validity and its relevance to an understanding of the nature of alcoholism would be in doubt. Clearly, it is necessary to demonstrate that results of classification help us to understand other facets of behavior as well, and these facets need to be related to the issue at hand.

Finally, other authors in this volume have emphasized the need for longitudinal research. I see an important application of classification research to longitudinal studies. The possibility that different personality types display different developmental trends in the addiction and treatment process needs to be explored. In this connection, causal modeling, which Huba and Bentler (1982) have used to study illicit drug use, could also be used in alcoholism research. Clearly, many other directions for classification research in alcohol use and abuse show potential for handsome dividends, particularly if some of the pitfalls that previous studies have encountered can be avoided.

References

Blashfield, R. K. "Propositions Regarding the Use of Cluster Analysis in Clinical Research." *Journal of Consulting and Clinical Psychology,* 1980, *48,* 456–459.

Canter, N., Smith, E. E., French, R., and Mezzich, J. "Psychiatric Diagnosis as Prototype Categorization." *Journal of Abnormal Psychology,* 1980, *89,* 181–193.

Clopton, J. R. "Alcoholism and the MMPI: A Review." *Journal of Studies on Alcohol,* 1978, *39,* 1540–1558.

Cox, W. M. "The Alcoholic's Personality: A Review of the Evidence." *Progress in Experimental Personality Research,* 1979, *9,* 89–148.

Donovan, D. M., Chaney, E. F., and O'Leary, M. R. "Alcoholic MMPI Subtypes: Relationship to Drinking Styles, Benefits, and Consequences." *Journal of Nervous and Mental Disease,* 1978, *166,* 553–561.

Gilberstadt, H., and Ducker, J. *A Handbook for Clinical and Actuarial MMPI Interpretation.* Philadelphia: Saunders, 1965.

Goldstein, S. G., and Linden, J. D. "Multivariate Classification of Alcoholics by Means of the MMPI." *Journal of Abnormal Psychology,* 1969, *74,* 661–669.

Huba, G. J., and Bentler, P. M. "A Developmental Theory of Drug Use: Derivation and Assessment of a Causal Modeling Approach." *Life Span Development and Behavior,* 1982, *4,* 147–203.

Jackson, D. N. "The Dynamics of Structured Personality Tests: 1971." *Psychological Review,* 1971, *78,* 229–248.

Jackson, D. N., and Carlson, K. A. "Convergent and Discriminant Validation of the Differential Personality Inventory." *Journal of Clinical Psychology,* 1973, *29,* 214–219.
Jackson, D. N., and Messick, S. *Differential Personality Inventory.* Cleveland, Ohio: Psychological Corporation, 1983.
Jackson, D. N., and Williams, D. R. "Occupational Classification in Terms of Interest Patterns." *Journal of Vocational Behavior,* 1975, *6,* 269–280.
Jellinek, E. M. "Phases in the Drinking History of Alcoholics." *Quarterly Journal of Studies in Alcohol,* 1946, *7,* 1–88.
Jellinek, E. M. *The Disease Concept of Alcoholism.* New Brunswick, N.J.: Hillhouse Press, 1960.
Lanyon, R. I. *A Handbook of MMPI Group Profiles.* Minneapolis: University of Minnesota Press, 1968.
Løberg, T. "MMPI-Based Personality Subtypes of Alcholics: Relationship to Drinking History, Psychometrics, and Neuropsychological Deficits." *Journal of Studies on Alcohol,* 1981, *42,* 766–782.
Marks, P. A., and Seeman, W. *Actuarial Description of Abnormal Personality: An Atlas for Use with the MMPI.* Baltimore: Williams and Wilkins, 1963.
Morey, L. C., and Blashfield, L. C. "Empirical Classification of Alcoholism: A Review." *Journal of Studies on Alcohol,* 1981, *42,* 925–937.
Paquin, M. J. R., and Jackson, D. N. "The Dimensionality of Psychopathology Descriptors." *Multivariate Behavioral Research,* 1981, *16,* 291–308.
Partington, J. T., and Johnson, F. G. "Personality Types Among Alcoholics." *Quarterly Journal of Studies on Alcohol,* 1969, *30,* 21–34.
Reed, P. L., and Jackson, D. N. "Clinical Judgment of Psychopathology: A Model for Inferential Accuracy." *Journal of Abnormal Psychology,* 1975, *84,* 475–482.
Skinner, H. A. "Assessment of Alcohol Problems: Basic Principles, Critical Issues, and Future Trends." In Y. Israel and others (Eds.), *Research Advances in Alcohol and Drug Problems.* Vol. 6. New York: Plenum, 1981.
Skinner, H. A., Jackson, D. N., Hoffman, H. "Alcoholic Personality Types: Identification and Correlates." *Journal of Abnormal Psychology,* 1974, *83,* 658–666.
Skinner, H. A., Reed, P. L., and Jackson, D. N. "Toward the Objective Diagnosis of Psychopathology: Generalizability of Modal Personality Profiles." *Journal of Consulting and Clinical Psychology,* 1976, *44,* 111–117.
Whitelock, R. P., Overall, J. E., and Patrick, J. H. "Personality Patterns and Alcohol Abuse in a State Hospital Population." *Journal of Abnormal Psychology,* 1971, *78,* 9–16.
Wiggins, J. S. *Personality and Prediction: Principles of Personality.* Reading, Mass.: Addison-Wesley, 1973.

Douglas N. Jackson has been senior professor of psychology at the University of Western Ontario, London, Canada, for the past eighteen years. He has held visiting positions at Educational Testing Service, Pennsylvania State University, University of Iowa, and Stanford University, where he studied alcohol problems with E. M. Jellinek and others. He has been active for a number of years in research on the assessment of psychopathology.

Index

C

D

E

F

G

H

I

J

K

N

O

P

R

S

T

U

V

W